Fractured Minds, Fractured Society

Understanding and Addressing the Mental Health Emergency in America

The HealthSpan Institute

Fractured Minds, Fractured Society:
Understanding and Addressing the Mental Health Emergency in
America

ISBN: 9798322412984

Printed in the United States of America

Contents

Chapter I:
Introduction

The Current State of Mental Health in America 7

The Impact of Untreated Mental Health Issues on Individuals and Society....................9

The Purpose and Structure of the Book....................11

Chapter II:
The Scope of the Mental Health Crisis

Prevalence of Mental Health Disorders in the USA 14

The Economic Burden of Mental Illness....................16

The Social and Cultural Factors Contributing to the Crisis....................19

Chapter III:
Barriers to Accessing Mental Health Care

Stigma and Misconceptions Surrounding Mental Health...22

Insufficient Mental Health Coverage in Insurance Plans.....25

Shortage of Mental Health Professionals....................29

Lack of Mental Health Education and Awareness................32

Chapter IV:
The Impact of Untreated Mental Health Issues

Consequences for Individuals 36

Consequences for Society 39

Chapter V:
Addressing the Mental Health Crisis:
A Multi-Faceted Approach

Increasing Access to Mental Health Services..........................43

Promoting Mental Health Education and Awareness..........46

Strengthening Community Support Systems 49

Chapter VI:
Innovations in Mental Health Treatment

The Role of Technology in Expanding Access to Care..........53

Emerging Therapies and Interventions 56

Chapter VII:
Addressing Mental Health Disparities

Mental Health Challenges in Underserved Communities...60

Culturally Sensitive Approaches to Mental
Health Treatment 63

Strategies for Reducing Mental Health Inequities................67

Chapter VIII:
The Role of Policy in
Transforming Mental Health Care

Advocating for Mental Health Parity Laws..............................71

Investing in Mental Health Research and Innovation..........74

Collaborating with Stakeholders to Develop Comprehensive
Mental Health Policies..78

Chapter IX:
Conclusion

Recap of Key Points and Recommendations 82

A Call to Action for Individuals, Communities, and
Policymakers 85

Resources

Mental Health Organizations and Support Groups 89

Recommended Reading and References 92

Glossary of Mental Health Terms 95

Chapter I: Introduction

The Current State of Mental Health in America

The United States is grappling with a mental health crisis of unprecedented proportions. In recent years, the nation has witnessed a disturbing surge in the prevalence of mental health disorders, affecting individuals from all walks of life. This alarming trend has far-reaching consequences, not only for those directly impacted but also for the fabric of American society as a whole.

According to the National Alliance on Mental Illness (NAMI), approximately one in five adults in the U.S. experiences mental illness each year [1]. This staggering statistic translates to nearly 50 million Americans struggling with mental health issues, ranging from anxiety and depression to more severe conditions such as bipolar disorder and schizophrenia. Even more concerning is the fact that these numbers have been steadily increasing over the past decade, with no signs of abating.

The mental health crisis is particularly acute among younger generations. A 2019 report by the American Psychological Association (APA) found that rates of depression, anxiety, and suicidal ideation have risen dramatically among adolescents and young adults in recent years [2]. This troubling trend is exemplified by the fact that suicide is now the second leading cause of death among individuals aged 10-34 in the United States [3].

The COVID-19 pandemic has only exacerbated the mental health crisis, as the nation grapples with the profound psychological impact of prolonged social isolation, economic uncertainty, and the loss of loved ones. A study conducted by the Kaiser Family Foundation found that during the pandemic, 40% of U.S. adults reported symptoms of anxiety or depressive disorder, a significant increase from the 10% reported prior to the outbreak [4].

The consequences of this mental health emergency extend far beyond the realm of personal well-being. Untreated mental health conditions can lead to a host of negative outcomes, including decreased productivity, increased healthcare costs, and strained relationships. Moreover, the stigma surrounding mental illness often prevents individuals from seeking the help they need, further perpetuating the cycle of suffering.

Despite the overwhelming evidence of a mental health crisis, the United States has struggled to mount an adequate response. Mental health services remain chronically underfunded and understaffed, with many individuals facing significant barriers to accessing the care they need. This is particularly true for marginalized communities, who often bear the brunt of the mental health burden while simultaneously facing the greatest obstacles to treatment.

The current state of mental health in America is a clarion call for action. It is imperative that we, as a society, recognize the urgency of this crisis and take decisive steps to address it. This will require a comprehensive, multi-faceted approach that encompasses increased funding for mental health services, the destigmatization of mental illness, and the development of innovative treatment modalities.

Only by confronting the mental health emergency head-on can we hope to build a more resilient, compassionate, and mentally healthy America. The time for action is now, and the stakes could not be higher.

References

1. National Alliance on Mental Illness. (2021). Mental Health By the Numbers. Retrieved from https://www.nami.org/mhstats
2. American Psychological Association. (2019). Stress in America: Generation Z. Retrieved from https://www.apa.org/news/press/releases/stress/2019/stress-america-2019.pdf
3. National Institute of Mental Health. (2021). Suicide. Retrieved from https://www.nimh.nih.gov/health/statistics/suicide
4. Kaiser Family Foundation. (2021). The Implications of COVID-19 for Mental Health and Substance Use. Retrieved from https://www.kff.org/coronavirus-covid-19/issue-brief/the-implications-of-covid-19-for-mental-health-and-substance-use/

The Impact of Untreated Mental Health Issues on Individuals and Society

The repercussions of untreated mental health conditions extend far beyond the personal struggles of affected individuals. When left unaddressed, mental health issues can have a profound and far-reaching impact on every aspect of a person's life, as well as on the broader societal landscape.

For individuals living with untreated mental health conditions, the consequences can be devastating. These individuals often experience a significant deterioration in their quality of life, as the symptoms of their condition interfere with their ability to function in daily life. They may struggle to maintain relationships, hold down a job, or pursue their educational goals. The constant battle with their own thoughts and emotions can be exhausting, leading to feelings of hopelessness and despair [1].

Moreover, untreated mental health issues can take a severe toll on an individual's physical health. Research has consistently shown that there is a strong link between mental and physical well-being. Individuals with untreated mental health conditions are at a higher risk of developing chronic physical health problems, such as heart disease, diabetes, and obesity [2]. This is due, in part, to the fact that mental health issues can lead to unhealthy behaviors, such as substance abuse, poor diet, and lack of exercise.

The impact of untreated mental health conditions extends beyond the individual, however. The ripple effects can be felt throughout society, as the consequences of these conditions strain relationships, communities, and social systems. Family members and loved ones often bear the brunt of this impact, as they struggle to support and care for their affected family member. This can lead to increased stress, financial burden, and emotional turmoil within the family unit [3].

In the workplace, untreated mental health issues can lead to decreased productivity, increased absenteeism, and higher rates of turnover. A study by the World Health Organization found that depression and anxiety disorders cost the global economy approximately $1 trillion in lost productivity each year [4]. This economic burden is felt not only by employers but also by society as a whole, as the costs of lost productivity and increased healthcare utilization are passed on to taxpayers and consumers.

The criminal justice system is another area where the impact of untreated mental health conditions is keenly felt. A significant proportion of individuals in the criminal justice system suffer from mental health issues, many of which are undiagnosed or untreated. This has led to a phenomenon known as the "criminalization of mental illness," where individuals with mental health conditions are more likely to be arrested, incarcerated, and subjected to violence within the criminal justice system [5].

Perhaps most tragically, untreated mental health conditions can lead to loss of life. Suicide, which is often the result of untreated depression or other mental health issues, is a leading cause of death worldwide. In the United States alone, there are approximately 130 suicides per day [6]. These deaths are a stark reminder of the devastating consequences of leaving mental health conditions untreated.

The impact of untreated mental health issues on individuals and society is a complex and multifaceted problem that requires urgent attention. By increasing access to mental health services, reducing stigma, and investing in prevention and early intervention, we can begin to mitigate the harmful effects of untreated mental illness. It is a public health imperative that we prioritize mental health as a society, recognizing that the well-being of our communities depends on the well-being of every individual within them.

References

1. National Alliance on Mental Illness. (2021). Mental Health Conditions. Retrieved from https://www.nami.org/About-Mental-Illness/Mental-Health-Conditions
2. Kolappa, K., Henderson, D. C., & Kishore, S. P. (2013). No physical health without mental health: lessons unlearned? Bulletin of the World Health Organization, 91(1), 3-3A. https://doi.org/10.2471/BLT.12.115063
3. Skundberg-Kletthagen, H., Wangensteen, S., Hall-Lord, M. L., & Hedelin, B. (2014). Relatives of patients with depression: experiences of everyday life. Scandinavian Journal of Caring Sciences, 28(3), 564-571. https://doi.org/10.1111/scs.12082
4. World Health Organization. (2019). Mental health in the workplace. Retrieved from https://www.who.int/teams/mental-health-and-substance-use/mental-health-in-the-workplace
5. Lamb, H. R., & Weinberger, L. E. (2005). The shift of psychiatric inpatient care from hospitals to jails and prisons. Journal of the American Academy of Psychiatry and the Law, 33(4), 529-534.
6. American Foundation for Suicide Prevention. (2021). Suicide Statistics. Retrieved from https://afsp.org/suicide-statistics/

The Purpose and Structure of the Book

In light of the alarming state of mental health in America and the far-reaching consequences of untreated mental illness, it is clear that urgent action is needed. This book, "Fractured Minds, Fractured Society: Understanding and Addressing the Mental Health Emergency in America," aims to contribute to the critical conversation surrounding mental health in the United States. By providing a comprehensive overview of the current crisis, exploring the factors that have contributed to its development, and proposing strategies for addressing it, this book seeks to inspire meaningful change in how we approach mental health as a society.

The purpose of this book is threefold. First, it aims to raise awareness about the severity and scale of the mental health crisis in America. By presenting a wealth of data, research, and personal narratives, the book illustrates the profound impact of mental illness on individuals, families, and communities across the nation. In doing so, it seeks to dispel the myths and misconceptions that have long surrounded mental health, and to underscore the urgent need for action.

Second, the book seeks to provide a nuanced understanding of the complex factors that have contributed to the current crisis. It explores the historical, social, economic, and cultural forces that have shaped our current mental health landscape, and examines how these forces intersect with issues of race, gender, and class. By situating the mental health crisis within a broader societal context, the book aims to foster a more comprehensive and empathetic understanding of the challenges we face.

Third, and perhaps most importantly, the book aims to offer a roadmap for addressing the mental health emergency in America. It presents a range of strategies and solutions, drawing on the latest research, best practices, and innovative approaches from across the globe. From increasing access to mental health services and reducing stigma, to investing in prevention and early intervention, the book explores a wide range of potential solutions. Ultimately, it argues that addressing the mental health crisis will require a collective effort, involving stakeholders from across the healthcare system, government, civil society, and beyond.

The structure of the book reflects these three core purposes. It is divided into three main sections, each of which builds upon the previous one to create a comprehensive and compelling narrative.

The first section, "Understanding the Crisis," provides an in-depth exploration of the current state of mental health in America. It examines the prevalence and impact of mental illness, the factors that have contributed to the current crisis, and the barriers that prevent individuals from accessing the care they need. Through a combination of data, research, and personal stories, this section paints a vivid picture of the challenges we face.

The second section, "Exploring the Solutions," presents a range of strategies and approaches for addressing the mental health crisis. It examines best practices from across the healthcare system, and explores innovative models for delivering mental health services. It also looks at the role of government, civil society, and other stakeholders in promoting mental health and well-being.

The final section, "Charting a Path Forward," offers a vision for a more mentally healthy America. It argues that addressing the mental health crisis will require a fundamental shift in how we think about and approach mental health as a society. It calls for a coordinated, collaborative effort that involves stakeholders from across the spectrum, and emphasizes the importance of prevention, early intervention, and community-based approaches.

Throughout the book, the writing style is engaging, accessible, and compelling. Complex ideas and data are presented in a clear and understandable way, making the book suitable for a wide range of readers. The use of personal narratives and case studies helps to humanize the issues and foster empathy and understanding.

Ultimately, "Fractured Minds, Fractured Society" is a call to action. It is a plea for us to confront the mental health emergency in America head-on, and to work together to build a society that values and promotes mental health and well-being for all. By providing a comprehensive understanding of the crisis and a roadmap for addressing it, this book aims to inspire the kind of collective action that is so urgently needed.

References

1. National Institute of Mental Health. (2021). Mental Illness. Retrieved from https://www.nimh.nih.gov/health/statistics/mental-illness
2. Substance Abuse and Mental Health Services Administration. (2021). Key Substance Use and Mental Health Indicators in the United States: Results from the 2020 National Survey on Drug Use and Health. Retrieved from https://www.samhsa.gov/data/report/2020-ns-duh-annual-national-report
3. [3] World Health Organization. (2018). Mental Health Atlas 2017. Retrieved from https://www.who.int/publications/i/item/9789241514019
4. [4] Patel, V., Saxena, S., Lund, C., Thornicroft, G., Baingana, F., Bolton, P., ... & UnÜtzer, J. (2018). The Lancet Commission on global mental health and sustainable development. The Lancet, 392(10157), 1553-1598. https://doi.org/10.1016/S0140-6736(18)31612-X

Chapter II:
The Scope of the Mental Health Crisis

Prevalence of Mental Health Disorders in the USA

The United States is facing an unprecedented mental health crisis, with a significant portion of the population grappling with mental health disorders. The prevalence of these conditions has reached alarming levels, affecting individuals from all walks of life and across all age groups. To truly comprehend the scope of this crisis, it is essential to delve into the data and statistics that reveal the extent of mental health disorders in America.

According to the National Institute of Mental Health (NIMH), an estimated 52.9 million adults in the United States, representing 21.0% of the adult population, experienced a mental illness in 2020 [1]. This staggering figure underscores the pervasiveness of mental health issues in the country. Among these individuals, 14.2 million adults, or 5.6% of the adult population, were diagnosed with a serious mental illness, which is defined as a mental, behavioral, or emotional disorder that substantially interferes with or limits one or more major life activities [1].

The prevalence of specific mental health disorders in the United States is equally concerning. Anxiety disorders, which include generalized anxiety disorder, panic disorder, and phobias, are the most common mental illnesses in the country. The NIMH estimates that 40 million adults in the U.S., or 19.1% of the adult population, had an anxiety disorder in the past year [2]. This means that nearly one in five adults in America experiences the debilitating symptoms of anxiety, such as excessive worry, restlessness, and difficulty concentrating.

Depression is another mental health disorder that affects a significant portion of the American population. In 2020, an estimated 21.0 million adults in the U.S., or 8.4% of the adult population, had at least one major depressive episode [1]. Depression can manifest in various ways, including persistent feelings of sadness, loss of interest in activities, changes in sleep and appetite, and thoughts of self-harm or suicide. The impact of depression on individuals and society is profound, as it can lead to decreased productivity, strained relationships, and a diminished quality of life.

Substance use disorders, which often co-occur with other mental health conditions, are also prevalent in the United States. In 2020, an estimated 40.3 million people aged 12 or older, or 14.5% of the population, had a substance use disorder in the past year [3]. This includes disorders related to the use of alcohol, illicit drugs, and prescription medications. Substance use disorders can have devastating consequences, including physical and mental health problems, social and legal issues, and an increased risk of overdose and death.

The prevalence of mental health disorders in the United States varies across different demographic groups. For example, women are more likely than men to experience anxiety and depression [1]. Young adults aged 18-25 have the highest prevalence of mental illness compared to other age groups, with 30.6% experiencing a mental illness in the past year [1]. Additionally, certain racial and ethnic minorities, such as American Indians and Alaska Natives, have higher rates of mental health disorders compared to the general population [4].

It is important to note that the prevalence of mental health disorders in the United States is likely underestimated due to various factors. These include the stigma associated with mental illness, which can prevent individuals from seeking help or disclosing their symptoms, as well as the lack of access to mental health services in certain communities. Furthermore, the COVID-19 pandemic has exacerbated the mental health crisis in America, with many individuals experiencing increased stress, anxiety, and depression due to the economic, social, and health-related challenges posed by the pandemic [5].

The high prevalence of mental health disorders in the United States underscores the urgent need for action. It is essential to prioritize mental health as a public health issue and to invest in prevention, early intervention, and treatment services. This includes increasing access to mental health care, reducing stigma and discrimination, and promoting mental health education and awareness. By addressing the prevalence of mental health disorders in America, we can work towards building a more resilient, compassionate, and mentally healthy society.

References

1. National Institute of Mental Health. (2021). Mental Illness. Retrieved from https://www.nimh.nih.gov/health/statistics/mental-illness
2. Anxiety and Depression Association of America. (2021). Facts & Statistics. Retrieved from https://adaa.org/understanding-anxiety/facts-statistics
3. Substance Abuse and Mental Health Services Administration. (2021). Key Substance Use and Mental Health Indicators in the United States: Results from the 2020 National Survey on Drug Use and Health. Retrieved from https://www.samhsa.gov/data/report/2020-nsduh-annual-national-report
4. American Psychiatric Association. (2017). Mental Health Disparities: Diverse Populations. Retrieved from https://www.psychiatry.org/psychiatrists/cultural-competency/education/mental-health-facts
5. Czeisler, M. É., Lane, R. I., Petrosky, E., Wiley, J. F., Christensen, A., Njai, R., ... & Rajaratnam, S. M. (2020). Mental health, substance use, and suicidal ideation during the COVID-19 pandemic—United States, June 24–30, 2020. Morbidity and Mortality Weekly Report, 69(32), 1049-1057. http://dx.doi.org/10.15585/mmwr.mm6932a1

The Economic Burden of Mental Illness

The prevalence of mental health disorders in the United States not only takes a toll on individuals and their loved ones but also has far-reaching economic consequences. The financial impact of mental illness is felt across various sectors, including healthcare, labor, and social services. As the nation grapples with the growing mental health crisis, it is crucial to understand the economic burden of these conditions and the urgent need for investment in prevention, treatment, and support services.

One of the most significant economic costs associated with mental illness is the increased healthcare expenditure. Individuals with mental health disorders often require ongoing medical care, including visits to mental health professionals, prescription medications, and hospitalization. According to a study published in the Journal of the American Medical Association, mental health conditions are among the most costly health conditions in the United States, with an estimated annual spending of $201 billion [1]. This figure accounts for both direct healthcare costs and indirect costs, such as lost productivity and reduced quality of life.

The economic burden of mental illness extends beyond the healthcare system, as these conditions can significantly impact an individual's ability to work and maintain employment. Mental health disorders are a leading cause of disability worldwide, and in the United States, they account for a substantial portion of lost workdays and reduced productivity [2]. The World Health Organization estimates that depression and anxiety disorders cost the global economy $1 trillion annually in lost productivity [3]. This loss is due to factors such as absenteeism, presenteeism (working while unwell), and reduced work performance.

Moreover, the economic impact of mental illness is not limited to the individuals directly affected by these conditions. Family members and caregivers often bear a significant financial burden, as they may need to reduce their own work hours or leave their jobs entirely to provide care and support. This can lead to a loss of income and increased expenses, such as the cost of transportation to medical appointments and the need for respite care services.

The social and economic costs of untreated mental health disorders can be particularly devastating. When individuals do not receive the care and support they need, their conditions may worsen over time, leading to more severe symptoms and a greater risk of disability. Untreated mental illness can also contribute to other social problems, such as homelessness, substance abuse, and involvement with the criminal justice system [4]. These issues not only have a profound impact on individuals and their communities but also place a significant strain on public resources and social services.

Investing in mental health services and support systems can help mitigate the economic burden of mental illness. Early intervention and treatment can prevent the progression of mental health disorders and reduce the need for more intensive and costly interventions down the line. Ensuring access to quality mental health care, including through the expansion of insurance coverage and the integration of mental health services into primary care settings, can help individuals receive the support they need to manage their conditions and maintain their overall well-being.

In addition to investing in treatment, promoting mental health education and awareness can help reduce the stigma associated with mental illness and encourage individuals to seek help early on. Workplace mental health initiatives, such as employee assistance programs and mental health training for managers, can create a supportive environment that promotes well-being and reduces the impact of mental health disorders on productivity and job retention.

The economic burden of mental illness in the United States is substantial and far-reaching. As the nation works to address the growing mental health crisis, it is essential to recognize the financial impact of these conditions and prioritize investment in prevention, treatment, and support services. By taking a proactive and comprehensive approach to mental health, we can not only improve the lives of individuals affected by these disorders but also strengthen the economic and social fabric of our communities.

References

1. Roehrig, C. (2016). Mental disorders top the list of the most costly conditions in the United States: $201 billion. Health Affairs, 35(6), 1130-1135. https://doi.org/10.1377/hlthaff.2015.1659
2. National Alliance on Mental Illness. (2021). Mental Health By the Numbers. Retrieved from https://www.nami.org/mhstats
3. World Health Organization. (2019). Mental health in the workplace. Retrieved from https://www.who.int/teams/mental-health-and-substance-use/mental-health-in-the-workplace
4. National Institute of Mental Health. (2021). Mental Illness. Retrieved from https://www.nimh.nih.gov/health/statistics/mental-illness
5. Substance Abuse and Mental Health Services Administration. (2021). Key Substance Use and Mental Health Indicators in the United States: Results from the 2020 National Survey on Drug Use and Health. Retrieved from https://www.samhsa.gov/data/report/2020-nsduh-annual-national-report

The Social and Cultural Factors Contributing to the Crisis

The mental health crisis in the United States is a complex and multifaceted issue that cannot be attributed to a single cause. While individual factors such as genetics and personal experiences play a role, it is crucial to recognize the broader social and cultural context that contributes to the development and exacerbation of mental health disorders. By examining these underlying factors, we can gain a deeper understanding of the current crisis and work towards creating a more supportive and mentally healthy society.

One of the most significant social factors contributing to the mental health crisis is the persistent stigma surrounding mental illness. Despite increased awareness and efforts to promote mental health education, negative attitudes and misconceptions about mental disorders remain prevalent in American society. Many individuals still view mental illness as a sign of weakness, a personal failing, or something to be ashamed of [1]. This stigma can prevent people from seeking help, disclosing their struggles, and accessing the support they need, leading to a worsening of their conditions over time.

The stigma associated with mental illness is often reinforced by cultural norms and expectations. In a society that values independence, self-reliance, and emotional restraint, admitting to mental health challenges can be seen as a violation of these norms. This is particularly true for certain demographic groups, such as men, who may feel pressure to adhere to traditional masculine stereotypes that discourage vulnerability and emotional expression [2]. Cultural attitudes towards mental health can also vary across different racial, ethnic, and religious communities, with some groups facing additional barriers to seeking help due to language differences, cultural beliefs, or mistrust of the healthcare system [3].

Another significant social factor contributing to the mental health crisis is the increasing pace and pressure of modern life. In recent decades, American society has undergone rapid changes, including technological advancements, globalization, and shifting economic and social landscapes. While these changes have brought many benefits, they have also created new sources of stress and challenges for individuals and communities. The rise of social media, for example, has been linked to increased rates of anxiety, depression, and loneliness, particularly among younger generations [4]. The constant connectivity and pressure to present a perfect image online can exacerbate feelings of inadequacy and social comparison, leading to mental health struggles.

The modern workplace has also become a significant source of stress and mental health challenges for many Americans. With longer work hours, increased job insecurity, and the blurring of boundaries between work and personal life, employees are facing unprecedented levels of pressure and burnout [5]. The culture of overwork and the glorification of hustle can make it difficult for individuals to prioritize their mental health and well-being, leading to a cycle of stress and exhaustion.

Socioeconomic factors, such as poverty, income inequality, and lack of access to resources, also play a crucial role in the mental health crisis. Individuals living in poverty or experiencing financial instability are at a higher risk of developing mental health disorders, as the stress and uncertainty of their circumstances can take a toll on their emotional well-being [6]. Additionally, marginalized communities, such as racial and ethnic minorities, LGBTQ+ individuals, and people with disabilities, often face unique stressors and barriers to accessing mental health services, leading to disparities in mental health outcomes [7].

The current political and social climate in the United States has also contributed to the mental health crisis. In recent years, the nation has experienced increasing levels of political polarization, social unrest, and divisive rhetoric. Exposure to constant news coverage of traumatic events, such as mass shootings, police brutality, and hate crimes, can have a profound impact on mental health, particularly for communities directly affected by these issues [8]. The sense of uncertainty and fear created by these events can exacerbate existing mental health conditions and contribute to the development of new ones.

Addressing the social and cultural factors contributing to the mental health crisis requires a multi-faceted approach that involves individuals, communities, and institutions. This includes promoting mental health education and awareness, challenging stigma and discrimination, and creating supportive environments that prioritize well-being. It also involves advocating for policies and programs that address the root causes of mental health disparities, such as poverty, racism, and lack of access to resources.

By recognizing and addressing the social and cultural factors that contribute to the mental health crisis, we can work towards creating a society that values and supports mental well-being for all individuals. This requires a collective effort to challenge harmful norms, promote compassion and understanding, and prioritize the mental health needs of our communities.

References

1. Parcesepe, A. M., & Cabassa, L. J. (2013). Public stigma of mental illness in the United States: a systematic literature review. Administration and Policy in Mental Health and Mental Health Services Research, 40(5), 384-399. https://doi.org/10.1007/s10488-012-0430-z
2. Addis, M. E., & Mahalik, J. R. (2003). Men, masculinity, and the contexts of help seeking. American Psychologist, 58(1), 5-14. https://doi.org/10.1037/0003-066X.58.1.5
3. Substance Abuse and Mental Health Services Administration. (2020). Double Jeopardy: COVID-19 and Behavioral Health Disparities for Black and Latino Communities in the U.S. Retrieved from https://www.samhsa.gov/sites/default/files/covid19-behavioral-health-disparities-black-latino-communities.pdf
4. Twenge, J. M., Joiner, T. E., Rogers, M. L., & Martin, G. N. (2018). Increases in depressive symptoms, suicide-related outcomes, and suicide rates among US adolescents after 2010 and links to increased new media screen time. Clinical Psychological Science, 6(1), 3-17. https://doi.org/10.1177/2167702617723376
5. World Health Organization. (2019). Mental health in the workplace. Retrieved from https://www.who.int/teams/mental-health-and-substance-use/mental-health-in-the-workplace
6. Sareen, J., Afifi, T. O., McMillan, K. A., & Asmundson, G. J. (2011). Relationship between household income and mental disorders: findings from a population-based longitudinal study. Archives of General Psychiatry, 68(4), 419-427. https://doi.org/10.1001/archgenpsychiatry.2011.15
7. American Psychiatric Association. (2017). Mental Health Disparities: Diverse Populations. Retrieved from https://www.psychiatry.org/psychiatrists/cultural-competency/education/mental-health-facts
8. Bor, J., Venkataramani, A. S., Williams, D. R., & Tsai, A. C. (2018). Police killings and their spillover effects on the mental health of black Americans: a population-based, quasi-experimental study. The Lancet, 392(10144), 302-310. https://doi.org/10.1016/S0140-6736(18)31130-9

Chapter III:
Barriers to Accessing Mental Health Care

Stigma and Misconceptions Surrounding Mental Health

One of the most significant barriers to addressing the mental health crisis in the United States is the persistent stigma and misconceptions that surround mental illness. Despite increased awareness and efforts to promote mental health education, negative attitudes and beliefs about mental disorders remain deeply entrenched in American society. These stigmas and misconceptions can have a profound impact on individuals living with mental health conditions, preventing them from seeking help, receiving support, and achieving recovery.

At the heart of the stigma surrounding mental illness is the idea that mental health disorders are a sign of weakness, a personal failing, or something to be ashamed of. This belief is rooted in a long history of misunderstanding and fear about mental illness, which has been perpetuated by media portrayals, cultural stereotypes, and a lack of accurate information [1]. Many people still view mental health conditions as fundamentally different from physical health problems, as if they are a reflection of an individual's character or moral fortitude rather than a legitimate medical issue.

One of the most harmful misconceptions about mental illness is the notion that people with mental health disorders are dangerous, unpredictable, or violent. This stereotype is often reinforced by sensationalized media coverage of rare instances of violence involving individuals with mental illness, which can lead to a distorted public perception of the risks associated with these conditions [2]. In reality, people with mental health disorders are far more likely to be victims of violence than perpetrators, and the vast majority of individuals with mental illness pose no threat to public safety [3].

Another common misconception is the idea that mental health disorders are not real illnesses, but rather a sign of personal weakness or a lack of willpower. This belief can lead to a dismissive attitude towards mental health struggles, with individuals being told to "snap out of it" or "just get over it" rather than receiving the compassion and support they need. This attitude fails to recognize the complex biological, psychological, and social factors that contribute to mental illness, and it can make individuals feel isolated, misunderstood, and reluctant to seek help.

The stigma surrounding mental illness can also intersect with other forms of discrimination and marginalization, such as racism, sexism, and homophobia. For example, research has shown that Black Americans are more likely to experience stigma related to mental health than white Americans, and they may face additional barriers to accessing mental health services due to cultural mistrust, lack of diversity among mental health providers, and other systemic inequities [4]. Similarly, LGBTQ+ individuals may encounter unique stressors and challenges that contribute to mental health struggles, but they may also face discrimination and lack of understanding from healthcare providers and social support systems [5].

The consequences of stigma and misconceptions surrounding mental health can be severe and far-reaching. When individuals internalize these negative beliefs, they may experience shame, self-doubt, and a reluctance to acknowledge their own mental health needs. This self-stigma can lead to delays in seeking treatment, poor adherence to treatment plans, and a reduced quality of life [6]. Additionally, the fear of being labeled or discriminated against can prevent individuals from disclosing their mental health struggles to friends, family members, or employers, leading to a lack of social support and accommodations that could improve their well-being.

Combating the stigma and misconceptions surrounding mental health requires a multi-faceted approach that involves education, awareness-raising, and cultural change. One key strategy is to promote accurate and compassionate media portrayals of mental illness, which can help to counter negative stereotypes and increase public understanding of these conditions [7]. This includes highlighting stories of recovery and resilience, as well as representing the diversity of individuals living with mental health disorders.

Another important approach is to increase mental health literacy and education, both among the general public and within healthcare and social service settings. This can involve providing training and resources to help individuals recognize the signs and symptoms of mental illness, understand the available treatment options, and know how to support loved ones who may be struggling [8]. It can also involve addressing the cultural and linguistic barriers that may prevent certain communities from accessing mental health information and services.

At a systemic level, addressing the stigma surrounding mental health requires a commitment to creating more inclusive and equitable policies and practices. This can involve advocating for mental health parity laws that ensure equal coverage for mental health services, as well as investing in community-based programs that promote mental wellness and resilience [9]. It can also involve addressing the social determinants of mental health, such as poverty, discrimination, and trauma, which can create additional barriers to care and support.

Ultimately, breaking down the stigma and misconceptions surrounding mental health is a critical step in addressing the mental health crisis in the United States. By promoting a more accurate, compassionate, and inclusive understanding of mental illness, we can create a society that values and supports the mental well-being of all individuals. This requires a collective effort to challenge harmful stereotypes, provide education and resources, and prioritize the mental health needs of our communities.

References

1. Corrigan, P. W., & Watson, A. C. (2002). Understanding the impact of stigma on people with mental illness. World Psychiatry, 1(1), 16-20.
2. McGinty, E. E., Webster, D. W., & Barry, C. L. (2013). Effects of news media messages about mass shootings on attitudes toward persons with serious mental illness and public support for gun control policies. American Journal of Psychiatry, 170(5), 494-501. https://doi.org/10.1176/appi.ajp.2013.13010014
3. Varshney, M., Mahapatra, A., Krishnan, V., Gupta, R., & Deb, K. S. (2016). Violence and mental illness: what is the true story? Journal of Epidemiology and Community Health, 70(3), 223-225. https://doi.org/10.1136/jech-2015-205546
4. Williams, D. R., González, H. M., Neighbors, H., Nesse, R., Abelson, J. M., Sweetman, J., & Jackson, J. S. (2007). Prevalence and distribution of major depressive disorder in African Americans, Caribbean blacks, and non-Hispanic whites: results from the National Survey of American Life. Archives of General Psychiatry, 64(3), 305-315. https://doi.org/10.1001/archpsyc.64.3.305
5. Meyer, I. H. (2003). Prejudice, social stress, and mental health in lesbian, gay, and bisexual populations: conceptual issues and research evidence. Psychological Bulletin, 129(5), 674-697. https://doi.org/10.1037/0033-2909.129.5.674
6. Corrigan, P. W., Druss, B. G., & Perlick, D. A. (2014). The impact of mental illness stigma on seeking and participating in mental health care. Psychological Science in the Public Interest, 15(2), 37-70. https://doi.org/10.1177/1529100614531398
7. Klin, A., & Lemish, D. (2008). Mental disorders stigma in the media: review of studies on production, content, and influences. Journal of Health Communication, 13(5), 434-449. https://doi.org/10.1080/10810730802198813
8. Jorm, A. F. (2012). Mental health literacy: empowering the community to take action for better mental health. American Psychologist, 67(3), 231-243. https://doi.org/10.1037/a0025957
9. Mechanic, D. (2002). Removing barriers to care among persons with psychiatric symptoms. Health Affairs, 21(3), 137-147. https://doi.org/10.1377/hlthaff.21.3.137

Insufficient Mental Health Coverage in Insurance Plans

One of the most significant barriers to accessing mental health care in the United States is the inadequate coverage of mental health services in many insurance plans. Despite the passage of the Mental Health Parity and Addiction Equity Act (MHPAEA) in 2008, which requires insurance companies to provide equal coverage for mental health and substance use disorder treatments as they do for medical and surgical care, disparities in coverage persist [1]. This lack of sufficient mental health coverage can have devastating consequences for individuals and families struggling with mental illness, forcing them to choose between paying out of pocket for necessary care or forgoing treatment altogether.

The issue of insufficient mental health coverage in insurance plans is rooted in a long history of discrimination and stigma surrounding mental illness. For decades, mental health conditions were viewed as distinct from physical health problems, and insurance companies often excluded or limited coverage for mental health services [2]. While the MHPAEA and the Affordable Care Act (ACA) have made significant strides in improving access to mental health care, loopholes and enforcement challenges have allowed many insurance plans to continue providing inadequate coverage.

One common way that insurance plans limit mental health coverage is through the use of higher copays, deductibles, and coinsurance rates for mental health services compared to medical and surgical care [3]. This means that even if an insurance plan nominally covers mental health treatment, the out-of-pocket costs for the individual can be prohibitively expensive. For example, an insurance plan may require a \$50 copay for a primary care visit but a \$100 copay for a therapy session, making it difficult for individuals to afford regular mental health care.

Another way that insurance plans restrict mental health coverage is by limiting the number of covered therapy sessions or hospital days for mental health treatment. While there may be no such limits on medical or surgical care, insurance plans often cap the number of mental health visits or days that they will cover in a given year [4]. This can be particularly problematic for individuals with severe or chronic mental illnesses who require ongoing, intensive treatment to manage their symptoms and prevent hospitalization.

Insurance plans may also exclude certain types of mental health providers or treatments from coverage. For instance, some plans may only cover mental health services provided by psychiatrists or psychologists, excluding other qualified mental health professionals such as licensed clinical social workers or marriage and family therapists [5]. This can limit the available pool of providers and make it more difficult for individuals to find a mental health professional who is covered by their insurance. Additionally, some plans may not cover newer or alternative treatments for mental illness, such as transcranial magnetic stimulation (TMS) or ketamine therapy, even when these treatments are medically necessary and recommended by a mental health provider [6].

The insufficient mental health coverage in many insurance plans can have serious consequences for individuals and society as a whole. When people are unable to access the mental health care they need, their conditions may worsen over time, leading to more severe symptoms, increased disability, and a greater risk of suicide [7]. Untreated mental illness can also have ripple effects on families, communities, and the economy, as individuals struggle to maintain relationships, employment, and overall functioning.

Moreover, the lack of adequate mental health coverage can exacerbate existing disparities in mental health care access and outcomes. Research has shown that racial and ethnic minorities, low-income individuals, and rural residents are more likely to face barriers to mental health care, including a lack of insurance coverage or difficulty finding providers who accept their insurance [8]. This can lead to worsening mental health disparities and a widening gap in access to care.

Addressing the issue of insufficient mental health coverage in insurance plans will require a multi-faceted approach that involves policy changes, advocacy, and education. One key strategy is to strengthen enforcement of the MHPAEA and close loopholes that allow insurance companies to provide unequal coverage for mental health services. This can involve increased oversight and penalties for non-compliance, as well as clearer guidance on what constitutes parity in coverage [9].

Another important approach is to expand the types of mental health providers and treatments that are covered by insurance plans. This can involve advocating for the inclusion of a wider range of qualified mental health professionals, such as licensed clinical social workers and marriage and family therapists, as well as coverage for evidence-based treatments that may be considered "non-traditional," such as TMS or ketamine therapy [10].

Additionally, increasing mental health literacy and education can help individuals understand their insurance coverage and advocate for their rights to access mental health care. This can involve providing resources and support to help people navigate complex insurance systems, as well as raising awareness about the importance of mental health parity and the consequences of untreated mental illness.

Ultimately, ensuring sufficient mental health coverage in insurance plans is a critical step in addressing the mental health crisis in the United States. By breaking down financial barriers to care and increasing access to a wide range of mental health services, we can create a more equitable and effective mental health care system that supports the well-being of all individuals and communities.

References

1. Mental Health Parity and Addiction Equity Act of 2008, Pub. L. No. 110-343, § 512, 122 Stat. 3765, 3881 (2008).
2. Appelbaum, P. S. (2006). The 'quiet' crisis in mental health services. Health Affairs, 25(5), 1205-1212. https://doi.org/10.1377/hlthaff.25.5.1205
3. National Alliance on Mental Illness. (2015). A long road ahead: Achieving true parity in mental health and substance use care. Retrieved from https://www.nami.org/Support-Education/Publications-Reports/Public-Policy-Reports/A-Long-Road-Ahead/2015-ALongRoadAhead
4. Goodell, S., Druss, B. G., & Walker, E. R. (2011). Mental disorders and medical comorbidity. Robert Wood Johnson Foundation. Retrieved from https://www.rwjf.org/en/library/research/2011/02/mental-disorders-and-medical-comorbidity.html
5. Bishop, T. F., Press, M. J., Keyhani, S., & Pincus, H. A. (2014). Acceptance of insurance by psychiatrists and the implications for access to mental health care. JAMA Psychiatry, 71(2), 176-181. https://doi.org/10.1001/jamapsychiatry.2013.2862
6. Gooding, G. (2020). Insurance Companies Still Don't Adequately Cover Mental Health Treatment. Verywell Mind. Retrieved from https://www.verywellmind.com/insurance-companies-still-dont-adequately-cover-mental-health-treatment-5091806
7. National Institute of Mental Health. (2021). Mental Illness. Retrieved from https://www.nimh.nih.gov/health/statistics/mental-illness
8. Patel, V., Burns, J. K., Dhingra, M., Tarver, L., Kohrt, B. A., & Lund, C. (2018). Income inequality and depression: a systematic review and meta-analysis of the association and a scoping review of mechanisms. World Psychiatry, 17(1), 76-89. https://doi.org/10.1002/wps.20492
9. Ali, M. M., Teich, J. L., & Mutter, R. (2017). Perceived unmet need for mental health and substance use treatment among adults with co-occurring disorders. Journal of Substance Abuse Treatment, 76, 63-72. https://doi.org/10.1016/j.jsat.2017.03.002
10. Ross, C., & Goldner, E. M. (2009). Stigma, negative attitudes and discrimination towards mental illness within the nursing profession: a review of the literature. Journal of Psychiatric and Mental Health Nursing, 16(6), 558-567. https://doi.org/10.1111/j.1365-2850.2009.01399.x

Shortage of Mental Health Professionals

One of the most pressing challenges in addressing the mental health crisis in the United States is the significant shortage of mental health professionals. As the demand for mental health services continues to rise, the supply of qualified providers has struggled to keep pace, leaving many individuals without access to the care they need. This shortage is particularly acute in certain regions and among specific populations, exacerbating existing disparities in mental health care access and outcomes.

The shortage of mental health professionals in the United States is a complex and multifaceted issue that stems from a variety of factors. One of the primary drivers is the aging of the mental health workforce, with many experienced providers nearing retirement age [1]. As these seasoned professionals leave the field, there are not enough new providers entering the pipeline to replace them, leading to a growing gap between supply and demand.

Another factor contributing to the shortage is the uneven distribution of mental health professionals across the country. While urban areas may have a relatively high concentration of providers, rural and underserved communities often struggle to attract and retain mental health professionals [2]. This geographic maldistribution can make it difficult for individuals in these areas to access care, even if they have insurance coverage or the means to pay for services.

The shortage of mental health professionals is also exacerbated by the limited diversity within the field. Research has shown that racial and ethnic minorities are significantly underrepresented among mental health providers, which can create barriers to care for individuals who prefer to work with a provider who shares their cultural background or language [3]. This lack of diversity can also contribute to cultural misunderstandings or biases in diagnosis and treatment, further widening mental health disparities.

The consequences of the shortage of mental health professionals are far-reaching and devastating. When individuals are unable to access the care they need, their mental health conditions may worsen over time, leading to more severe symptoms, increased disability, and a greater risk of suicide [4]. The shortage can also lead to longer wait times for appointments, which can be particularly problematic for individuals in crisis or those with acute symptoms that require immediate attention.

Moreover, the shortage of mental health professionals can place a significant burden on the providers who are currently working in the field. With high caseloads and limited resources, many mental health professionals are at risk of burnout, which can lead to decreased quality of care and high turnover rates [5]. This can further exacerbate the shortage, as burned-out providers leave the field and discourage others from entering it.

Addressing the shortage of mental health professionals will require a comprehensive and sustained effort that involves multiple stakeholders, including policymakers, educational institutions, professional organizations, and healthcare systems. One key strategy is to invest in the training and education of the next generation of mental health providers, with a focus on increasing diversity and cultural competence [6]. This can involve providing scholarships and loan forgiveness programs to attract a wider range of individuals to the field, as well as developing curricula that prioritize cultural sensitivity and humility.

Another important approach is to improve the distribution of mental health professionals across the country, particularly in underserved and rural areas. This can involve offering incentives, such as tax breaks or student loan repayment programs, to encourage providers to practice in these communities [7]. It can also involve expanding the use of telehealth and other technology-based solutions to bridge the gap between providers and patients in remote areas.

Additionally, addressing the shortage of mental health professionals will require a broader shift in how we value and prioritize mental health care in the United States. This can involve advocating for increased funding for mental health services, as well as working to reduce the stigma surrounding mental illness and seeking help [8]. By creating a culture that prioritizes mental health and well-being, we can attract more individuals to the field and ensure that everyone has access to the care they need.

The shortage of mental health professionals is a critical barrier to addressing the mental health crisis in the United States. Without a sufficient number of qualified providers, many individuals will continue to fall through the cracks, unable to access the care and support they need to manage their mental health conditions. Addressing this shortage will require a multi-faceted approach that involves increasing the diversity and cultural competence of the mental health workforce, improving the geographic distribution of providers, and prioritizing mental health care as a societal value. Only by taking bold and sustained action can we hope to build a mental health care system that truly meets the needs of all individuals and communities.

References

1. Figley, C. R., & Figley, K. R. (2017). A wave of departures: The coming crisis in mental health care. Psychological Injury and Law, 10(4), 307-315. https://doi.org/10.1007/s12207-017-9302-x
2. Fortney, J. C., Harman, J. S., Xu, S., & Dong, F. (2010). The association between rural residence and the use, type, and quality of depression care. The Journal of Rural Health, 26(3), 205-213. https://doi.org/10.1111/j.1748-0361.2010.00290.x
3. Holley, L. C., & Tavassoli, K. Y. (2015). The role of cultural competence in mental health service use among racial and ethnic minorities. Administration and Policy in Mental Health and Mental Health Services Research, 42(6), 671-682. https://doi.org/10.1007/s10488-015-0642-0
4. National Institute of Mental Health. (2021). Mental Illness. Retrieved from https://www.nimh.nih.gov/health/statistics/mental-illness
5. Morse, G., Salyers, M. P., Rollins, A. L., Monroe-DeVita, M., & Pfahler, C. (2012). Burnout in mental health services: A review of the problem and its remediation. Administration and Policy in Mental Health and Mental Health Services Research, 39(5), 341-352. https://doi.org/10.1007/s10488-011-0352-1
6. Alegría, M., Alvarez, K., & DiMarzio, K. (2017). Immigration and mental health. Current Epidemiology Reports, 4(2), 145-155. https://doi.org/10.1007/s40471-017-0111-2
7. Watanabe-Galloway, S., Madison, L., Watkins, K. L., Nguyen, A. T., & Chen, L. (2015). Recruitment and retention of mental health care providers in rural Nebraska: perceptions of providers and administrators. Rural and Remote Health, 15(4), 3392. https://doi.org/10.22605/RRH3392
8. Henderson, C., Evans-Lacko, S., & Thornicroft, G. (2013). Mental illness stigma, help seeking, and public health programs. American Journal of Public Health, 103(5), 777-780. https://doi.org/10.2105/AJPH.2012.301056

Lack of Mental Health Education and Awareness

One of the most significant barriers to addressing the mental health crisis in the United States is the widespread lack of mental health education and awareness. Despite the high prevalence of mental health disorders and the devastating impact they can have on individuals, families, and communities, there remains a profound gap in public understanding about mental illness, its causes, and the available treatment options. This lack of knowledge and awareness can have far-reaching consequences, perpetuating stigma, preventing individuals from seeking help, and hindering efforts to improve mental health care access and quality.

The lack of mental health education and awareness in the United States is rooted in a long history of misunderstanding and neglect surrounding mental illness. For centuries, mental health conditions were viewed as a sign of moral weakness or personal failing, rather than a legitimate medical issue requiring compassionate care and support [1]. While scientific understanding of mental illness has advanced significantly in recent decades, public attitudes and beliefs have been slower to evolve, leaving many individuals and communities without the knowledge and resources they need to prioritize mental health and well-being.

One of the most problematic aspects of the lack of mental health education and awareness is the persistence of stigma and misconceptions surrounding mental illness. Many people continue to view mental health conditions as a source of shame or embarrassment, rather than a common and treatable health issue [2]. This stigma can manifest in a variety of ways, from overt discrimination and social exclusion to more subtle forms of bias and misunderstanding. For example, individuals with mental illness may be viewed as dangerous, unpredictable, or incapable of leading fulfilling lives, despite evidence to the contrary [3].

The lack of mental health education and awareness can also prevent individuals from recognizing the signs and symptoms of mental illness in themselves or others. Without a basic understanding of what constitutes normal vs. abnormal mental health, many people may struggle to identify when they or a loved one are in need of help [4]. This can lead to delays in seeking treatment, which can allow mental health conditions to worsen over time and become more difficult to manage.

Even when individuals do recognize the need for mental health care, the lack of education and awareness can create barriers to accessing appropriate services. Many people may be unsure of where to turn for help, or may not realize that effective treatments are available [5]. Others may be hesitant to seek care due to concerns about cost, confidentiality, or the perceived stigma associated with mental health treatment. Without a clear understanding of the mental health care system and the resources available to them, individuals and families may struggle to navigate the complex landscape of services and support.

The lack of mental health education and awareness is particularly problematic among certain populations and communities that have historically been underserved by the mental health care system. For example, racial and ethnic minorities, LGBTQ+ individuals, and those living in rural or low-income areas may face additional barriers to accessing mental health care, including language and cultural differences, limited provider availability, and systemic inequities [6]. Without targeted outreach and education efforts, these communities may remain isolated from the resources and support they need to prioritize mental health and well-being.

Addressing the lack of mental health education and awareness will require a comprehensive and sustained effort that involves multiple stakeholders, including policymakers, educators, healthcare providers, and community organizations. One key strategy is to integrate mental health education into existing educational curricula, beginning in early childhood and continuing through high school and beyond [7]. By providing age-appropriate information about mental health and well-being, we can help young people develop the knowledge, skills, and attitudes they need to prioritize their own mental health and support others in need.

Another important approach is to expand public awareness campaigns and outreach efforts, particularly in communities that have been historically marginalized or underserved. This can involve partnering with trusted community leaders and organizations to deliver culturally sensitive and linguistically appropriate information about mental health and available resources [8]. It can also involve leveraging social media and other digital platforms to reach a wider audience and combat misinformation and stigma.

Healthcare providers also have a critical role to play in promoting mental health education and awareness. By integrating mental health screening and education into routine primary care visits, providers can help identify individuals at risk for mental health conditions and connect them with appropriate services and support [9]. They can also serve as trusted sources of information and guidance, helping patients and families navigate the complex mental health care system and make informed decisions about treatment options.

Ultimately, addressing the lack of mental health education and awareness will require a fundamental shift in how we think about and prioritize mental health in the United States. By providing individuals and communities with the knowledge, skills, and resources they need to support mental health and well-being, we can begin to break down the barriers that prevent so many from accessing the care and support they need. This will require a sustained commitment from all sectors of society, but the potential benefits – in terms of improved health outcomes, increased productivity, and greater social cohesion – are well worth the investment.

References

1. Farreras, I. G. (2019). History of mental illness. In R. Biswas-Diener & E. Diener (Eds.), Noba textbook series: Psychology. Champaign, IL: DEF Publishers. Retrieved from http://noba.to/65w3s7ex

2. Corrigan, P. W., & Watson, A. C. (2002). Understanding the impact of stigma on people with mental illness. World Psychiatry, 1(1), 16-20. Retrieved from https://www.ncbi.nlm.nih.gov/pmc/articles/PMC1489832/

3. Pescosolido, B. A. (2013). The public stigma of mental illness: What do we think; what do we know; what can we prove? Journal of Health and Social Behavior, 54(1), 1-21. https://doi.org/10.1177/0022146512471197

4. Jorm, A. F. (2012). Mental health literacy: Empowering the community to take action for better mental health. American Psychologist, 67(3), 231-243. https://doi.org/10.1037/a0025957

5. Gulliver, A., Griffiths, K. M., & Christensen, H. (2010). Perceived barriers and facilitators to mental health help-seeking in young people: a systematic review. BMC Psychiatry, 10,

113. https://doi.org/10.1186/1471-244X-10-113

6. Substance Abuse and Mental Health Services Administration. (2020). Double Jeopardy: COVID-19 and Behavioral Health Disparities for Black and Latino Communities in the U.S. Retrieved from https://www.samhsa.gov/sites/default/files/covid19-behavioral-health-disparities-black-latino-communities.pdf

7. Kutcher, S., Wei, Y., Costa, S., Gusmão, R., Skokauskas, N., & Sourander, A. (2016). Enhancing mental health literacy in young people. European Child & Adolescent Psychiatry, 25(6), 567-569. https://doi.org/10.1007/s00787-016-0867-9

8. Watkins, D. C., & Jefferson, S. O. (2013). Recommendations for the use of online social support for African American men. Psychological Services, 10(3), 323-332. https://doi.org/10.1037/a0027904

9. Ojeda, V. D., & McGuire, T. G. (2006). Gender and racial/ethnic differences in use of outpatient mental health and substance use services by depressed adults. Psychiatric Quarterly, 77(3), 211-222. https://doi.org/10.1007/s11126-006-9008-9

Chapter IV: The Impact of Untreated Mental Health Issues

Consequences for Individuals

The impact of untreated mental health issues on individuals can be profound and far-reaching, affecting every aspect of their lives. When mental health conditions are left unaddressed, they can lead to a cascade of negative consequences that can erode an individual's quality of life, relationships, and overall well-being. These consequences can be particularly devastating for those who are already vulnerable, such as individuals living in poverty, those with chronic health conditions, and members of marginalized communities.

One of the most immediate and tangible consequences of untreated mental health issues is a decreased quality of life. Mental health conditions such as depression, anxiety, and post-traumatic stress disorder (PTSD) can cause intense emotional distress, making it difficult for individuals to find joy and meaning in their daily lives [1]. They may struggle to engage in activities they once enjoyed, withdraw from social interactions, and experience a pervasive sense of hopelessness or helplessness. Over time, these symptoms can lead to a vicious cycle of isolation and despair, further exacerbating the underlying mental health condition.

Untreated mental health issues can also take a significant toll on an individual's physical health. Research has consistently shown that there is a strong link between mental and physical well-being, with mental health conditions increasing the risk of developing chronic health problems such as heart disease, diabetes, and obesity [2]. This is due in part to the fact that individuals with untreated mental health issues may engage in unhealthy behaviors, such as smoking, substance abuse, and neglecting self-care, as a way of coping with their emotional distress. Additionally, the chronic stress and inflammation associated with mental health conditions can have a direct impact on physical health, weakening the immune system and increasing the risk of disease [3].

Another devastating consequence of untreated mental health issues is the increased risk of suicide. Suicide is a leading cause of death worldwide, and individuals with mental health conditions are at a significantly higher risk of suicide than the general population [4]. In fact, studies have shown that up to 90% of individuals who die by suicide have a diagnosable mental health condition at the time of their death [5]. The risk of suicide is particularly high for individuals with untreated depression, bipolar disorder, and substance use disorders, but any mental health condition can increase the risk if left unaddressed.

Untreated mental health issues can also have a profound impact on an individual's relationships and social functioning. Mental health conditions can cause individuals to withdraw from friends and family, struggle to communicate effectively, and engage in behaviors that strain or damage their relationships [6]. For example, an individual with untreated depression may become irritable, lash out at loved ones, or neglect important social obligations, leading to conflicts and misunderstandings. Over time, these strained relationships can lead to a sense of loneliness and isolation, further exacerbating the underlying mental health condition.

In addition to the personal consequences, untreated mental health issues can also have significant implications for an individual's professional life. Mental health conditions can impair cognitive functioning, making it difficult for individuals to concentrate, make decisions, and perform at their best [7]. They may struggle to meet deadlines, communicate effectively with colleagues, or maintain a consistent work schedule, leading to decreased productivity and job performance. In some cases, untreated mental health issues can even lead to job loss or long-term unemployment, further compounding the financial and emotional stress on the individual and their family.

The consequences of untreated mental health issues can be particularly severe for individuals from marginalized communities, who often face additional barriers to accessing care and support. For example, racial and ethnic minorities may experience discrimination, language barriers, and cultural stigma that prevent them from seeking help for mental health concerns [8]. LGBTQ+ individuals may face rejection, violence, and minority stress that exacerbate mental health issues and make it difficult to access affirming care [9]. Individuals living in poverty may struggle to afford mental health treatment or may prioritize other basic needs over their own well-being.

Addressing the consequences of untreated mental health issues will require a multi-faceted approach that includes increasing access to affordable, culturally competent care, reducing stigma and discrimination, and promoting mental health education and awareness. It will also require a fundamental shift in how we think about and prioritize mental health as a society, recognizing that mental well-being is essential to overall health and quality of life.

By investing in prevention, early intervention, and comprehensive treatment for mental health conditions, we can help individuals avoid the devastating consequences of untreated mental illness and lead fulfilling, productive lives. This will require a coordinated effort from policymakers, healthcare providers, educators, and community leaders, but the potential benefits – in terms of improved health outcomes, increased productivity, and greater social cohesion – are well worth the investment.

References

1. Rapaport, M. H., Clary, C., Fayyad, R., & Endicott, J. (2005). Quality-of-life impairment in depressive and anxiety disorders. American Journal of Psychiatry, 162(6), 1171-1178. https://doi.org/10.1176/appi.ajp.162.6.1171
2. Katon, W. J. (2003). Clinical and health services relationships between major depression, depressive symptoms, and general medical illness. Biological Psychiatry, 54(3), 216-226. https://doi.org/10.1016/S0006-3223(03)00273-7
3. Slavich, G. M., & Irwin, M. R. (2014). From stress to inflammation and major depressive disorder: a social signal transduction theory of depression. Psychological Bulletin, 140(3), 774-815. https://doi.org/10.1037/a0035302

4. World Health Organization. (2021). Suicide. Retrieved from https://www.who.int/news-room/fact-sheets/detail/suicide
5. Cavanagh, J. T., Carson, A. J., Sharpe, M., & Lawrie, S. M. (2003). Psychological autopsy studies of suicide: a systematic review. Psychological Medicine, 33(3), 395-405. https://doi.org/10.1017/S0033291702006943
6. Hammen, C., & Brennan, P. A. (2002). Interpersonal dysfunction in depressed women: impairments independent of depressive symptoms. Journal of Affective Disorders, 72(2), 145-156. https://doi.org/10.1016/S0165-0327(01)00455-4
7. Lerner, D., & Henke, R. M. (2008). What does research tell us about depression, job performance, and work productivity? Journal of Occupational and Environmental Medicine, 50(4), 401-410. https://doi.org/10.1097/JOM.0b013e31816bae50
8. Substance Abuse and Mental Health Services Administration. (2020). Double Jeopardy: COVID-19 and Behavioral Health Disparities for Black and Latino Communities in the U.S. Retrieved from https://www.samhsa.gov/sites/default/files/covid19-behavioral-health-disparities-black-latino-communities.pdf
9. Meyer, I. H. (2003). Prejudice, social stress, and mental health in lesbian, gay, and bisexual populations: conceptual issues and research evidence. Psychological Bulletin, 129(5), 674-697. https://doi.org/10.1037/0033-2909.129.5.674

Consequences for Society

The impact of untreated mental health issues extends far beyond the individuals who suffer from them. When left unaddressed, mental health conditions can have a ripple effect on society as a whole, leading to a range of negative consequences that strain our healthcare systems, economy, and social fabric. These consequences are often overlooked or underestimated, but they have real and measurable costs that affect us all.

One of the most significant consequences of untreated mental health issues for society is the increased burden on our healthcare systems. When individuals with mental health conditions do not receive timely and appropriate care, their symptoms can worsen over time, leading to more severe and complex problems that require more intensive and costly interventions [1]. For example, individuals with untreated depression may develop chronic physical health problems, such as heart disease or diabetes, that require ongoing medical treatment and hospitalization. Similarly, individuals with untreated substance use disorders may experience more frequent and severe overdoses, requiring emergency medical care and long-term rehabilitation.

The costs associated with these increased healthcare needs are staggering. A report by the National Alliance on Mental Illness (NAMI) estimated that untreated mental health conditions cost the U.S. economy over $300 billion annually in lost productivity, healthcare expenses, and disability benefits [2]. These costs are borne not only by the individuals and families affected by mental illness but also by taxpayers and society as a whole through increased insurance premiums, reduced economic output, and strain on public resources.

In addition to the direct healthcare costs, untreated mental health issues can also have a significant impact on the workforce and economy. Mental health conditions are a leading cause of disability worldwide, and they can impair an individual's ability to work, learn, and participate fully in society [3]. When individuals with mental health conditions are unable to access appropriate care and support, they may struggle to maintain employment, leading to reduced productivity, absenteeism, and high turnover rates. This not only affects the individuals and their families but also has ripple effects on businesses and the broader economy.

The economic costs of untreated mental health issues are particularly concerning given the current state of the U.S. workforce. A report by the World Health Organization (WHO) estimated that depression and anxiety disorders cost the global economy over $1 trillion annually in lost productivity [4]. In the United States, where mental health conditions are particularly prevalent, these costs are even higher. A study by the American Heart Association estimated that workplace stress alone costs the U.S. economy over $300 billion annually in lost productivity, healthcare expenses, and employee turnover [5].

Beyond the economic costs, untreated mental health issues can also have a profound impact on public safety and the criminal justice system. Research has consistently shown that individuals with untreated mental health conditions are at a higher risk of becoming involved with the criminal justice system, either as perpetrators or victims of crime [6]. This is due in part to the fact that untreated mental health conditions can impair judgment, impulse control, and decision-making, leading to behaviors that may be illegal or dangerous.

The consequences of this increased involvement with the criminal justice system are devastating for individuals, families, and communities. Incarceration can exacerbate existing mental health conditions, leading to further deterioration and increased risk of suicide [7]. It can also disrupt family relationships, leading to increased rates of child welfare involvement and intergenerational trauma. Moreover, the costs associated with incarceration and criminal justice involvement are enormous, draining public resources that could be better spent on prevention, treatment, and support services.

Addressing the societal consequences of untreated mental health issues will require a comprehensive and coordinated approach that involves multiple sectors and stakeholders. This includes investing in prevention and early intervention services, such as school-based mental health programs and community outreach initiatives, to identify and address mental health concerns before they escalate [8]. It also includes expanding access to affordable, high-quality mental health treatment, including through the integration of mental health services into primary care settings and the use of technology-based interventions.

Perhaps most importantly, addressing the societal consequences of untreated mental health issues will require a fundamental shift in how we think about and prioritize mental health as a society. This includes challenging the stigma and discrimination that prevent individuals from seeking help, and promoting a culture of compassion, understanding, and support for those affected by mental illness. It also includes recognizing that mental health is essential to overall health and well-being, and that investing in mental health is not only a moral imperative but also a sound economic and social policy.

The consequences of untreated mental health issues for society are vast and far-reaching, affecting our healthcare systems, economy, and social fabric in profound and lasting ways. By investing in prevention, treatment, and support services, and by promoting a culture of compassion and understanding, we can mitigate these consequences and build a stronger, more resilient society for all. The costs of inaction are simply too high to ignore.

References

1. National Institute of Mental Health. (2021). Mental Illness. Retrieved from https://www.nimh.nih.gov/health/statistics/mental-illness
2. National Alliance on Mental Illness. (2021). Mental Health By the Numbers. Retrieved from https://www.nami.org/mhstats
3. World Health Organization. (2021). Mental disorders. Retrieved from https://www.who.int/news-room/fact-sheets/detail/mental-disorders
4. World Health Organization. (2019). Mental health in the workplace. Retrieved from https://www.who.int/teams/mental-health-and-substance-use/mental-health-in-the-workplace
5. American Heart Association. (2021). Resilience in the Workplace: An Evidence Review and Implications for Practice. Retrieved from https://www.heart.org/en/healthy-living/healthy-lifestyle/mental-health-and-wellbeing/resilience-in-the-workplace-an-evidence-review-and-implications-for-practice
6. Fazel, S., & Seewald, K. (2012). Severe mental illness in 33,588 prisoners worldwide: systematic review and meta-regression analysis. British Journal of Psychiatry, 200(5), 364-373. https://doi.org/10.1192/bjp.bp.111.096370
7. Fazel, S., Ramesh, T., & Hawton, K. (2017). Suicide in prisons: an international study of prevalence and contributory factors. The Lancet Psychiatry, 4(12), 946-952. https://doi.org/10.1016/S2215-0366(17)30430-3
8. Durlak, J. A., & Wells, A. M. (1997). Primary prevention mental health programs for children and adolescents: A meta-analytic review. American Journal of Community Psychology, 25(2), 115-152. https://doi.org/10.1023/A:1024654026646

Chapter V: Addressing the Mental Health Crisis: A Multi-Faceted Approach

Increasing Access to Mental Health Services

One of the most critical steps in addressing the mental health crisis in the United States is increasing access to mental health services. Despite the high prevalence of mental health conditions and the devastating consequences of untreated mental illness, many individuals struggle to access the care and support they need. This is due to a range of barriers, including cost, insurance coverage, provider shortages, and stigma, that prevent individuals from seeking and receiving timely and appropriate mental health treatment.

Expanding insurance coverage for mental health services is a key strategy for increasing access to care. The Affordable Care Act (ACA) made significant strides in this direction by requiring most health plans to cover mental health and substance use disorder services at parity with medical and surgical benefits [1]. This means that insurance companies cannot impose higher copays, deductibles, or visit limits on mental health services than they do for other types of care. However, despite these protections, many individuals still face barriers to accessing covered services, such as high out-of-pocket costs or limited provider networks.

To truly expand access to mental health services, it is essential to strengthen enforcement of mental health parity laws and close loopholes that allow insurance companies to limit coverage. This includes increasing oversight and penalties for non-compliant plans, as well as educating consumers about their rights and how to appeal denied claims [2]. It also includes advocating for policies that expand coverage for a wider range of mental health services, such as case management, peer support, and community-based interventions, that are essential for promoting recovery and well-being.

In addition to expanding insurance coverage, increasing access to mental health services will require investing in the mental health workforce. The United States currently faces a severe shortage of mental health professionals, particularly in rural and underserved areas [3]. This shortage is projected to worsen in the coming years as the demand for mental health services continues to grow and many current providers reach retirement age. To address this shortage, it is essential to invest in the recruitment, training, and retention of a diverse and culturally competent mental health workforce.

This can include providing loan forgiveness and scholarship programs to attract students to mental health professions, particularly those from underrepresented backgrounds [4]. It can also include expanding the scope of practice for non-physician providers, such as psychologists, social workers, and peer support specialists, who can provide high-quality mental health services in a variety of settings [5]. Additionally, investing in the use of technology, such as telepsychiatry and mobile health applications, can help bridge the gap between providers and patients in underserved areas and expand access to care [6].

Another key strategy for increasing access to mental health services is integrating mental health care into primary care settings. Primary care providers are often the first point of contact for individuals with mental health concerns, and they play a critical role in identifying and treating common mental health conditions, such as depression and anxiety [7]. By integrating mental health screening, assessment, and treatment into routine primary care visits, providers can help reduce stigma, improve early identification and intervention, and provide more comprehensive and coordinated care.

Collaborative care models, which involve close coordination between primary care providers and mental health specialists, have been shown to be particularly effective in improving outcomes for individuals with mental health conditions [8]. These models typically involve a primary care provider, a care manager, and a psychiatric consultant working together to develop and implement a treatment plan tailored to the individual's needs and preferences. By providing mental health services in a familiar and trusted setting, collaborative care can help reduce barriers to care and improve engagement and adherence to treatment.

Increasing access to mental health services will also require addressing the social and economic determinants of mental health, such as poverty, housing instability, and discrimination. Research has consistently shown that individuals who experience these social and economic stressors are at higher risk of developing mental health conditions and face greater barriers to accessing care [9]. To truly promote mental health and well-being, it is essential to invest in policies and programs that address these underlying determinants, such as affordable housing, living wages, and anti-discrimination protections.

Finally, increasing access to mental health services will require a fundamental shift in how we think about and prioritize mental health as a society. This includes challenging the stigma and misconceptions that prevent individuals from seeking help, and promoting a culture of openness, compassion, and support for those affected by mental illness. It also includes recognizing that mental health is essential to overall health and well-being, and that investing in mental health services is not only a moral imperative but also a sound public health and economic policy.

The mental health crisis in the United States is a complex and multifaceted problem that requires a comprehensive and sustained effort to address. By increasing access to mental health services through expanding insurance coverage, investing in the mental health workforce, integrating mental health care into primary care settings, addressing social and economic determinants of mental health, and promoting a culture of compassion and support, we can begin to turn the tide on this crisis and build a more resilient and mentally healthy society for all.

References

1. United States Department of Labor. (2021). Mental Health and Substance Use Disorder Parity. Retrieved from https://www.dol.gov/agencies/ebsa/laws-and-regulations/laws/mental-health-and-substance-use-disorder-parity
2. National Alliance on Mental Illness. (2021). What is Mental Health Parity? Retrieved from https://www.nami.org/Your-Journey/Individuals-with-Mental-Illness/Understanding-Health-Insurance/What-is-Mental-Health-Parity
3. Health Resources and Services Administration. (2021). Behavioral Health Workforce Projections, 2017-2030. Retrieved from https://bhw.hrsa.gov/sites/default/files/bureau-health-workforce/data-research/behavioral-health-workforce-projections-fact-sheet.pdf
4. American Psychological Association. (2021). Workforce Development and Retention. Retrieved from https://www.apa.org/advocacy/workforce-development
5. Substance Abuse and Mental Health Services Administration. (2021). Behavioral Health Workforce. Retrieved from https://www.samhsa.gov/workforce
6. American Psychiatric Association. (2021). Telepsychiatry. Retrieved from https://www.psychiatry.org/psychiatrists/practice/telepsychiatry
7. Katon, W. J. (2003). Clinical and health services relationships between major depression, depressive symptoms, and general medical illness. Biological Psychiatry, 54(3), 216-226. https://doi.org/10.1016/S0006-3223(03)00273-7
8. Archer, J., Bower, P., Gilbody, S., Lovell, K., Richards, D., Gask, L., Dickens, C., & Coventry, P. (2012). Collaborative care for depression and anxiety problems. Cochrane Database of Systematic Reviews, 10. https://doi.org/10.1002/14651858.CD006525.pub2
9. Allen, J., Balfour, R., Bell, R., & Marmot, M. (2014). Social determinants of mental health. International Review of Psychiatry, 26(4), 392-407. https://doi.org/10.3109/09540261.2014.928270

Promoting Mental Health Education and Awareness

In addition to increasing access to mental health services, promoting mental health education and awareness is a crucial component of addressing the mental health crisis in the United States. Despite the high prevalence of mental health conditions, there remains a significant lack of understanding and awareness about mental health among the general public. This lack of knowledge can perpetuate stigma, prevent individuals from seeking help, and contribute to the marginalization and discrimination of those with mental health conditions.

Implementing mental health literacy programs in schools is one key strategy for promoting mental health education and awareness. Mental health literacy refers to the knowledge, attitudes, and beliefs that individuals have about mental health and mental illness [1]. By providing age-appropriate education about mental health topics, such as emotional regulation, stress management, and help-seeking behaviors, schools can help young people develop the skills and knowledge they need to maintain their own mental health and support others who may be struggling.

Effective mental health literacy programs in schools should be comprehensive, evidence-based, and culturally responsive. They should be integrated into the curriculum at all grade levels and should involve a range of stakeholders, including teachers, administrators, counselors, and families [2]. By starting mental health education early and reinforcing it throughout a student's academic career, schools can help normalize discussions about mental health, reduce stigma, and promote a culture of wellness and support.

Encouraging open dialogue about mental health in the workplace is another important strategy for promoting mental health education and awareness. Mental health conditions are a leading cause of disability and absenteeism in the workplace, and they can have significant impacts on productivity, morale, and overall organizational health [3]. However, many employees are reluctant to disclose their mental health conditions or seek support due to fear of stigma, discrimination, or negative career consequences.

To create a mentally healthy workplace, employers should prioritize mental health education and awareness as part of their overall wellness strategy. This can include providing training for managers and supervisors on how to recognize and respond to signs of mental health distress, as well as offering employee assistance programs and other resources for those who may be struggling [4]. Employers should also work to create a culture of openness and support, where employees feel safe and comfortable discussing their mental health needs and seeking help when necessary.

Leveraging media and technology to combat stigma is another key strategy for promoting mental health education and awareness. Media portrayals of mental illness have historically been negative, sensationalized, and inaccurate, contributing to public misunderstanding and fear about mental health conditions [5]. However, media and technology can also be powerful tools for promoting accurate and compassionate representations of mental health and reducing stigma.

One promising approach is to engage individuals with lived experience of mental illness as media spokespeople and content creators. By sharing their stories and perspectives, these individuals can help humanize mental illness, challenge stereotypes, and provide hope and inspiration to others who may be struggling [6]. Social media platforms, in particular, offer opportunities for individuals to connect with others who share their experiences, access credible information and resources, and engage in advocacy and awareness-raising efforts.

Technology can also be leveraged to deliver mental health education and support directly to individuals, particularly those who may face barriers to accessing traditional mental health services. Mobile apps, online self-help programs, and virtual therapy platforms can provide accessible, convenient, and cost-effective ways for individuals to learn about mental health, develop coping skills, and connect with mental health professionals [7]. However, it is important to ensure that these technologies are evidence-based, user-friendly, and appropriate for diverse populations.

Promoting mental health education and awareness will require a sustained and collaborative effort from a range of stakeholders, including policymakers, educators, employers, healthcare providers, and media professionals. It will also require a fundamental shift in how we think about and prioritize mental health as a society. This includes recognizing that mental health is an essential component of overall health and well-being, and that promoting mental health literacy and reducing stigma are critical public health priorities.

By investing in mental health education and awareness, we can create a society where individuals feel empowered to seek help when they need it, where mental health is discussed openly and honestly, and where those with mental health conditions are treated with dignity, respect, and compassion. Ultimately, promoting mental health education and awareness is not only the right thing to do, but it is also a smart investment in the health, productivity, and well-being of our communities and our nation as a whole.

References

1. Kutcher, S., Wei, Y., & Coniglio, C. (2016). Mental health literacy: Past, present, and future. The Canadian Journal of Psychiatry, 61(3), 154-158. https://doi.org/10.1177/0706743715616609
2. Kutcher, S., Wei, Y., & Morgan, C. (2015). Successful application of a Canadian mental health curriculum resource by usual classroom teachers in significantly and sustainably improving student mental health literacy. The Canadian Journal of Psychiatry, 60(12), 580-586. https://doi.org/10.1177/070674371506001209
3. World Health Organization. (2019). Mental health in the workplace. Retrieved from https://www.who.int/teams/mental-health-and-substance-use/mental-health-in-the-workplace
4. Center for Workplace Mental Health. (2021). Workplace Mental Health. Retrieved from http://workplacementalhealth.org/
5. McGinty, E. E., Kennedy-Hendricks, A., Choksy, S., & Barry, C. L. (2016). Trends in news media coverage of mental illness in the United States: 1995-2014. Health Affairs, 35(6), 1121-1129. https://doi.org/10.1377/hlthaff.2016.0011
6. Marino, C., Child, B., & Campbell Krasinski, V. (2016). Sharing experience learned firsthand (SELF): Self-disclosure of lived experience in mental health services and supports. Psychiatric Rehabilitation Journal, 39(2), 154-160. https://doi.org/10.1037/prj0000171
7. Lattie, E. G., Adkins, E. C., Winquist, N., Stiles-Shields, C., Wafford, Q. E., & Graham, A. K. (2019). Digital mental health interventions for depression, anxiety, and enhancement of psychological well-being among college students: Systematic review. Journal of Medical Internet Research, 21(7), e12869. https://doi.org/10.2196/12869

Strengthening Community Support Systems

While increasing access to mental health services and promoting mental health education and awareness are critical components of addressing the mental health crisis, it is equally important to focus on strengthening community support systems. Community support systems refer to the network of relationships, resources, and services that individuals can draw upon to maintain their mental health and well-being. These systems can include family and friends, peer support groups, faith-based organizations, community centers, and other local institutions that provide a sense of belonging, purpose, and support.

Developing peer support programs is one promising strategy for strengthening community support systems. Peer support refers to the provision of emotional, social, and practical assistance by individuals who have experienced mental health challenges themselves [1]. Peer support can take many forms, including one-on-one mentoring, group support meetings, and online forums or chat rooms. By connecting with others who have faced similar struggles, individuals can gain valuable insights, coping strategies, and a sense of empowerment and hope.

Peer support programs have been shown to be effective in improving mental health outcomes, increasing social connectedness, and reducing hospitalization and crisis service use [2]. They can also help to reduce stigma and discrimination by demonstrating that recovery and resilience are possible. To be effective, peer support programs should be culturally responsive, trauma-informed, and integrated with other mental health services and supports.

Collaborating with faith-based organizations is another important strategy for strengthening community support systems. Faith-based organizations, such as churches, synagogues, mosques, and temples, play a vital role in the lives of many individuals and communities. They can provide a sense of meaning, purpose, and social connection, as well as practical support and resources in times of need. Faith-based organizations can also be important partners in promoting mental health education and awareness, reducing stigma, and connecting individuals to mental health services and supports.

Effective collaboration with faith-based organizations requires building trust, respect, and understanding between mental health professionals and faith leaders [3]. It also requires recognizing and valuing the unique strengths and perspectives that faith-based organizations bring to the table, while also ensuring that mental health services are evidence-based and culturally appropriate. By working together, mental health professionals and faith-based organizations can create a more seamless and holistic system of care that addresses the spiritual, emotional, and social needs of individuals and communities.

Engaging family members and caregivers in the treatment process is another critical component of strengthening community support systems. Family members and caregivers are often the first to notice changes in a loved one's mental health and the first to provide support and encouragement. However, they can also experience significant stress, burden, and emotional distress themselves, particularly if they lack the knowledge, skills, and resources to effectively support their loved one's recovery.

Engaging family members and caregivers in the treatment process can help to reduce their stress and improve their own mental health and well-being, while also improving outcomes for the individual with mental illness [4]. This can involve providing education and training on mental health conditions, treatment options, and coping strategies, as well as offering support groups and counseling services specifically for family members and caregivers. It can also involve actively involving family members and caregivers in treatment planning and decision-making, and recognizing and valuing their unique insights and perspectives.

Strengthening community support systems will require a collaborative and integrated approach that involves a range of stakeholders, including mental health professionals, community organizations, faith-based institutions, schools, employers, and policymakers. It will also require a shift in how we think about mental health and well-being, recognizing that they are not just individual responsibilities but collective ones that require the support and engagement of entire communities.

By investing in peer support programs, collaborating with faith-based organizations, engaging family members and caregivers, and building strong and resilient community support systems, we can create a society where individuals feel connected, supported, and empowered to maintain their mental health and well-being. Ultimately, strengthening community support systems is not only an essential component of addressing the mental health crisis, but it is also a fundamental building block of a healthy, thriving, and compassionate society.

References

1. Davidson, L., Bellamy, C., Guy, K., & Miller, R. (2012). Peer support among persons with severe mental illnesses: A review of evidence and experience. World Psychiatry, 11(2), 123-128. https://doi.org/10.1016/j.wpsyc.2012.05.009
2. Chinman, M., George, P., Dougherty, R. H., Daniels, A. S., Ghose, S. S., Swift, A., & Delphin-Rittmon, M. E. (2014). Peer support services for individuals with serious mental illnesses: Assessing the evidence. Psychiatric Services, 65(4), 429-441. https://doi.org/10.1176/appi.ps.201300244
3. Milstein, G., Manierre, A., & Yali, A. M. (2010). Psychological care for persons of diverse religions: A collaborative continuum. Professional Psychology: Research and Practice, 41(5), 371-381. https://doi.org/10.1037/a0021074
4. Dixon, L. B., Holoshitz, Y., & Nossel, I. (2016). Treatment engagement of individuals experiencing mental illness: Review and update. World Psychiatry, 15(1), 13-20. https://doi.org/10.1002/wps.20306
5. Substance Abuse and Mental Health Services Administration. (2016). Creating a healthier life: A step-by-step guide to wellness. Retrieved from https://store.samhsa.gov/product/Creating-a-Healthier-Life-/SMA16-4958
6. National Alliance on Mental Illness. (2021). Family members and caregivers. Retrieved from https://www.nami.org/Your-Journey/Family-Members-and-Caregivers
7. American Psychological Association. (2021). Building community resilience to disaster. Retrieved from https://www.apa.org/advocacy/building-community-resilience

Chapter VI: Innovations in Mental Health Treatment

The Role of Technology in Expanding Access to Care

In recent years, technology has emerged as a powerful tool for expanding access to mental health care and support. From teletherapy platforms to mobile mental health apps, technology is transforming the way we deliver and receive mental health services. By leveraging the power of digital tools, we can overcome many of the barriers that have traditionally prevented individuals from seeking or receiving care, such as stigma, cost, and geographic isolation.

One of the most promising applications of technology in mental health is the use of teletherapy and online counseling services. Teletherapy refers to the delivery of mental health services via video conferencing, phone, or chat platforms, allowing individuals to connect with mental health professionals from the comfort and privacy of their own homes [1]. This can be particularly beneficial for individuals who live in rural or underserved areas, who have mobility or transportation challenges, or who simply prefer the convenience and flexibility of online therapy.

Research has shown that teletherapy can be just as effective as in-person therapy for a range of mental health conditions, including depression, anxiety, and post-traumatic stress disorder [2]. In fact, some studies have found that clients may be more likely to open up and engage in therapy when they feel more comfortable and in control of their environment. Teletherapy can also help to reduce the stigma associated with seeking mental health care, as individuals can access services discreetly and on their own terms.

Mobile mental health apps are another promising application of technology in expanding access to care. Mental health apps can provide a wide range of tools and resources, such as mood tracking, guided meditations, cognitive-behavioral therapy exercises, and peer support forums [3]. These apps can be particularly useful for individuals who may not have access to traditional mental health services, who are looking for additional support between therapy sessions, or who prefer a self-guided approach to managing their mental health.

While the quality and effectiveness of mental health apps can vary widely, there is growing evidence to suggest that they can be a useful adjunct to traditional therapy or a standalone intervention for mild to moderate mental health concerns [4]. However, it is important to ensure that mental health apps are evidence-based, user-friendly, and appropriate for diverse populations, and that they are integrated with other mental health services and supports.

In addition to teletherapy and mental health apps, technology is also being used to support mental health research and innovation. Artificial intelligence and machine learning, for example, are being used to analyze large datasets and identify patterns and risk factors for mental health conditions [5]. This can help researchers to develop more targeted and effective interventions, as well as to identify individuals who may be at high risk for developing mental health problems.

Technology is also being used to create more immersive and engaging mental health interventions, such as virtual reality exposure therapy for phobias and anxiety disorders [6]. By creating realistic and controlled virtual environments, therapists can help individuals to confront and overcome their fears in a safe and gradual manner. Virtual reality interventions have been shown to be effective for a range of mental health conditions, and may be particularly useful for individuals who have difficulty engaging in traditional exposure therapy.

While the use of technology in mental health care holds great promise, it is important to recognize that it is not a panacea and that there are potential limitations and risks to consider. For example, not all individuals may have access to the necessary technology or digital literacy skills to engage in teletherapy or use mental health apps effectively. There are also concerns about the privacy and security of personal health information shared through digital platforms, as well as the potential for technology to exacerbate existing disparities in mental health care access and outcomes.

To ensure that technology is used effectively and equitably to expand access to mental health care, it will be important to invest in digital infrastructure and training, to develop and enforce appropriate regulations and standards, and to prioritize the needs and preferences of diverse communities. It will also be important to integrate technology-based interventions with other mental health services and supports, such as in-person therapy, peer support, and community-based resources.

Ultimately, the role of technology in expanding access to mental health care is an exciting and rapidly evolving area that holds great promise for improving the lives of individuals and communities affected by mental health conditions. By leveraging the power of digital tools and innovations, we can create a more accessible, affordable, and effective mental health care system that meets the diverse needs of all individuals.

References

1. American Psychological Association. (2020). What is telepsychology? Retrieved from https://www.apa.org/practice/guidelines/telepsychology
2. Brenes, G. A., Ingram, C. W., & Danhauer, S. C. (2011). Benefits and challenges of conducting psychotherapy by telephone. Professional Psychology: Research and Practice, 42(6), 543-549. https://doi.org/10.1037/a0026135
3. Torous, J., & Roberts, L. W. (2017). The ethical use of mobile health technology in clinical psychiatry. Journal of Nervous and Mental Disease, 205(1), 4-8. https://doi.org/10.1097/NMD.0000000000000596
4. Firth, J., Torous, J., Nicholas, J., Carney, R., Pratap, A., Rosenbaum, S., & Sarris, J. (2017). The efficacy of smartphone-based mental health interventions for depressive symptoms: A meta-analysis of randomized controlled trials. World Psychiatry, 16(3), 287-298. https://doi.org/10.1002/wps.20472
5. Shatte, A. B. R., Hutchinson, D. M., & Teague, S. J. (2019). Machine learning in mental health: A scoping review of methods and applications. Psychological Medicine, 49(9), 1426-1448. https://doi.org/10.1017/S0033291719000151
6. Maples-Keller, J. L., Bunnell, B. E., Kim, S. J., & Rothbaum, B. O. (2017). The use of virtual reality technology in the treatment of anxiety and other psychiatric disorders. Harvard Review of Psychiatry, 25(3), 103-113. https://doi.org/10.1097/HRP.0000000000000138

7. Hilty, D. M., Ferrer, D. C., Parish, M. B., Johnston, B., Callahan, E. J., & Yellowlees, P. M. (2013). The effectiveness of telemental health: A 2013 review. Telemedicine and e-Health, 19(6), 444-454. https://doi.org/10.1089/tmj.2013.0075

Emerging Therapies and Interventions

As our understanding of mental health continues to evolve, so too do the therapies and interventions available to individuals seeking treatment. While traditional approaches such as cognitive-behavioral therapy and medication management remain the mainstay of mental health care, there is a growing interest in exploring new and innovative treatments that can complement or even replace these established methods. From mindfulness-based therapies to cutting-edge neurostimulation techniques, these emerging approaches offer the potential for more targeted, personalized, and effective mental health care.

One of the most promising areas of innovation in mental health treatment is the use of mindfulness-based therapies. Mindfulness refers to the practice of bringing one's attention to the present moment with openness, curiosity, and non-judgment [1]. By cultivating mindfulness skills, individuals can learn to better regulate their emotions, reduce stress and anxiety, and improve their overall well-being.

Mindfulness-based therapies, such as mindfulness-based stress reduction (MBSR) and mindfulness-based cognitive therapy (MBCT), have been shown to be effective for a range of mental health conditions, including depression, anxiety, and post-traumatic stress disorder [2]. These therapies typically involve a combination of meditation, yoga, and other mindfulness practices, as well as group discussion and individual support.

One of the key advantages of mindfulness-based therapies is that they can be easily integrated into daily life and practiced independently, making them a accessible and sustainable option for long-term mental health management. Additionally, mindfulness-based therapies have been shown to have few side effects and can be used safely in combination with other treatments, such as medication or traditional therapy.

Another area of innovation in mental health treatment is the use of neurostimulation techniques, such as transcranial magnetic stimulation (TMS) and deep brain stimulation (DBS). These techniques involve the use of targeted electrical or magnetic stimulation to modulate brain activity and alleviate symptoms of mental health conditions.

TMS, for example, uses a magnetic coil placed near the scalp to stimulate specific areas of the brain that are thought to be involved in mood regulation [3]. This non-invasive technique has been FDA-approved for the treatment of depression and has shown promise for other conditions such as anxiety and obsessive-compulsive disorder.

DBS, on the other hand, involves the surgical implantation of electrodes into specific areas of the brain, which are then stimulated with precise electrical pulses [4]. While more invasive than TMS, DBS has shown promise for the treatment of severe and treatment-resistant cases of depression, as well as other neurological conditions such as Parkinson's disease.

While neurostimulation techniques are still considered experimental for many mental health conditions, they offer the potential for more targeted and individualized treatment approaches that can address the underlying neural mechanisms of these disorders. As research in this area continues to evolve, it is likely that we will see even more advanced and refined neurostimulation techniques emerge in the coming years.

Perhaps one of the most exciting and controversial areas of innovation in mental health treatment is the use of psychedelic-assisted psychotherapy. This approach involves the use of psychedelic substances, such as psilocybin (found in "magic mushrooms"), LSD, and MDMA, in combination with traditional psychotherapy to treat a range of mental health conditions.

While the use of psychedelics in mental health treatment is still highly regulated and controversial, there is a growing body of research suggesting that these substances can be effective for conditions such as depression, anxiety, and post-traumatic stress disorder [5]. The therapeutic effects of psychedelics are thought to be mediated by their ability to promote neuroplasticity, enhance emotional processing, and facilitate profound insights and spiritual experiences.

Psychedelic-assisted psychotherapy typically involves a series of sessions in which the patient ingests a carefully controlled dose of the psychedelic substance under the guidance and supervision of a trained therapist. The patient then engages in a process of self-exploration and insight, often accompanied by music and other sensory stimuli designed to enhance the therapeutic experience.

While the use of psychedelics in mental health treatment is still in the early stages of research and development, many experts believe that these substances have the potential to revolutionize the field of mental health care. As more studies are conducted and regulatory barriers are overcome, it is possible that psychedelic-assisted psychotherapy could become a more widely available and accepted treatment option in the future.

As exciting as these emerging therapies and interventions are, it is important to approach them with caution and careful consideration. Many of these techniques are still in the early stages of research and development, and their long-term safety and efficacy have yet to be fully established. Additionally, these approaches may not be appropriate or effective for everyone, and it is important to work closely with a qualified mental health professional to determine the best course of treatment for an individual's unique needs and circumstances.

Nonetheless, the emergence of these innovative therapies and interventions offers hope and promise for the future of mental health care. By expanding the range of available treatment options and approaches, we can better meet the diverse needs of individuals seeking mental health support and improve outcomes for those living with mental health conditions. As research in this area continues to evolve, it is likely that we will see even more groundbreaking and transformative innovations emerge in the years to come.

References

1. Kabat-Zinn, J. (2003). Mindfulness-based interventions in context: Past, present, and future. Clinical Psychology: Science and Practice, 10(2), 144-156. https://doi.org/10.1093/clipsy.bpg016
2. Khoury, B., Lecomte, T., Fortin, G., Masse, M., Therien, P., Bouchard, V., Chapleau, M.-A., Paquin, K., & Hofmann, S. G. (2013). Mindfulness-based therapy: A comprehensive meta-analysis. Clinical Psychology Review, 33(6), 763-771. https://doi.org/10.1016/j.cpr.2013.05.005
3. Lefaucheur, J.-P., Aleman, A., Baeken, C., Benninger, D. H., Brunelin, J., Di Lazzaro, V., Filipović, S. R., Grefkes, C., Hasan, A., Hummel, F. C., Jääskeläinen, S. K., Langguth, B., Leocani, L., Londero, A., Nardone, R., Nguyen, J.-P., Nyffeler, T., Oliveira-Maia, A. J., Oliviero, A., ... Ziemann, U. (2020). Evidence-based guidelines on the therapeutic use of repetitive transcranial magnetic stimulation (rTMS): An update (2014-2018). Clinical Neurophysiology, 131(2), 474-528. https://doi.org/10.1016/j.clinph.2019.11.002
4. Youngerman, B. E., & Youngerman, S. (2019). Deep brain stimulation for treatment-resistant depression. American Journal of Psychiatry Residents' Journal, 14(4), 4-7. https://doi.org/10.1176/appi.ajp-rj.2019.140402
5. Reiff, C. M., Richman, E. E., Nemeroff, C. B., Carpenter, L. L., Widge, A. S., Rodriguez, C. I., Kalin, N. H., McDonald, W. M., & the Work Group on Biomarkers and Novel Treatments, a Division of the American Psychiatric Association Council of Research. (2020). Psychedelics and psychedelic-assisted psychotherapy. American Journal of Psychiatry, 177(5), 391-410. https://doi.org/10.1176/appi.ajp.2019.19010035

Chapter VII: Addressing Mental Health Disparities

Mental Health Challenges in Underserved Communities

The mental health crisis in the United States is a complex and multifaceted issue that affects individuals from all walks of life. However, certain communities face unique challenges and barriers when it comes to accessing mental health care and support. These underserved communities, which include racial and ethnic minorities, low-income individuals, and those living in rural areas, often experience higher rates of mental health disorders and face significant disparities in access to and quality of care.

One of the most pressing mental health challenges facing underserved communities is the lack of culturally competent care. Cultural competence refers to the ability of healthcare providers to deliver care that is responsive to the unique cultural, linguistic, and social needs of diverse patient populations [1]. Unfortunately, many mental health providers lack the training and experience necessary to provide culturally competent care, which can lead to misdiagnosis, inappropriate treatment, and poor outcomes for patients from diverse backgrounds.

For example, studies have shown that African Americans are more likely to receive a misdiagnosis of schizophrenia compared to white patients with similar symptoms, due in part to cultural biases and stereotypes held by healthcare providers [2]. Similarly, Asian Americans may be less likely to seek mental health treatment due to cultural stigma and a lack of culturally appropriate services, leading to underdiagnosis and undertreatment of mental health conditions in this population [3].

Another significant challenge facing underserved communities is the lack of access to mental health services. Many low-income and rural communities have a shortage of mental health providers, particularly those who accept Medicaid or other public insurance plans [4]. This can make it difficult for individuals in these communities to find affordable and accessible mental health care, even if they recognize the need for treatment.

Moreover, even when mental health services are available in underserved communities, they may not be tailored to the specific needs and preferences of the population. For example, many mental health interventions are developed and tested on predominantly white, middle-class populations and may not be effective or appropriate for individuals from diverse cultural backgrounds or with limited English proficiency [5].

The consequences of these mental health disparities can be devastating for individuals and communities. Untreated mental health conditions can lead to a range of negative outcomes, including increased risk of chronic physical health problems, substance abuse, unemployment, homelessness, and involvement with the criminal justice system [6]. These outcomes can perpetuate cycles of poverty and marginalization, further exacerbating mental health disparities and limiting opportunities for social and economic mobility.

Addressing the mental health challenges facing underserved communities will require a comprehensive and collaborative approach that involves multiple sectors and stakeholders. One key strategy is to invest in the training and recruitment of a diverse and culturally competent mental health workforce. This can involve providing cultural competency training for existing providers, as well as supporting the education and advancement of mental health professionals from diverse backgrounds [7].

Another important approach is to expand access to mental health services in underserved communities through the use of innovative delivery models and technologies. For example, telepsychiatry and mobile health interventions can help to bridge the gap between providers and patients in rural and remote areas, while community health workers and peer support specialists can provide culturally appropriate outreach and support in hard-to-reach communities [8].

It is also essential to address the social determinants of mental health in underserved communities, such as poverty, discrimination, and trauma. This can involve advocating for policies and programs that promote economic stability, social inclusion, and community resilience, as well as partnering with community-based organizations and leaders to develop culturally relevant interventions and support systems [9].

Ultimately, addressing the mental health challenges facing underserved communities will require a fundamental shift in how we think about and prioritize mental health equity in the United States. This means recognizing that mental health is not just an individual issue, but a social and political one that is deeply intertwined with issues of race, class, and power. It means investing in the mental health and well-being of all communities, particularly those that have been historically marginalized and underserved. And it means working together to build a more just and equitable society that values the dignity and humanity of all individuals, regardless of their background or circumstances.

The mental health challenges facing underserved communities are complex and deeply entrenched, but they are not insurmountable. By taking a holistic and culturally responsive approach to mental health care, and by working collaboratively across sectors and communities, we can begin to close the gap in mental health disparities and ensure that everyone has access to the care and support they need to thrive. It will not be easy, but it is a moral and social imperative that we cannot afford to ignore.

References

1. Substance Abuse and Mental Health Services Administration. (2014). Improving Cultural Competence. Treatment Improvement Protocol (TIP) Series No. 59. HHS Publication No. (SMA) 14-4849. https://store.samhsa.gov/sites/default/files/d7/priv/sma14-4849.pdf
2. Schwartz, R. C., & Blankenship, D. M. (2014). Racial disparities in psychotic disorder diagnosis: A review of empirical literature. World Journal of Psychiatry, 4(4), 133-140. https://doi.org/10.5498/wjp.v4.i4.133

3. Sue, S., Cheng, J. K. Y., Saad, C. S., & Chu, J. P. (2012). Asian American mental health: A call to action. American Psychologist, 67(7), 532-544. https://doi.org/10.1037/a0028900
4. Cummings, J. R., Allen, L., Clennon, J., Ji, X., & Druss, B. G. (2017). Geographic access to specialty mental health care across high- and low-income US communities. JAMA Psychiatry, 74(5), 476-484. https://doi.org/10.1001/jamapsychiatry.2017.0303
5. Alegría, M., Alvarez, K., Ishikawa, R. Z., DiMarzio, K., & McPeck, S. (2016). Removing obstacles to eliminating racial and ethnic disparities in behavioral health care. Health Affairs, 35(6), 991-999. https://doi.org/10.1377/hlthaff.2016.0029
6. Eack, S. M., & Newhill, C. E. (2012). Racial disparities in mental health outcomes after psychiatric hospital discharge among individuals with severe mental illness. Social Work Research, 36(1), 41-52. https://doi.org/10.1093/swr/svs014
7. American Psychological Association. (2017). Multicultural Guidelines: An Ecological Approach to Context, Identity, and Intersectionality. https://www.apa.org/about/policy/multicultural-guidelines.pdf
8. Barnett, M. L., Ray, K. N., Souza, J., & Mehrotra, A. (2018). Trends in telemedicine use in a large commercially insured population, 2005-2017. JAMA, 320(20), 2147-2149. https://doi.org/10.1001/jama.2018.12354
9. Alegría, M., NeMoyer, A., Falgàs Bagué, I., Wang, Y., & Alvarez, K. (2018). Social Determinants of Mental Health: Where We Are and Where We Need to Go. Current Psychiatry Reports, 20(11), 95. https://doi.org/10.1007/s11920-018-0969-9

Culturally Sensitive Approaches to Mental Health Treatment

As the United States becomes increasingly diverse, it is more important than ever to develop and implement culturally sensitive approaches to mental health treatment. Cultural sensitivity refers to the ability of healthcare providers to recognize, understand, and respect the unique cultural beliefs, values, and practices of their patients and to adapt their treatment approaches accordingly [1]. By embracing cultural sensitivity, mental health providers can improve the quality and effectiveness of care for individuals from diverse backgrounds and help to reduce disparities in mental health outcomes.

One of the key principles of culturally sensitive mental health treatment is the recognition that culture plays a significant role in shaping an individual's understanding and experience of mental health and illness. Different cultures may have different beliefs about the causes and nature of mental health problems, as well as different expectations for treatment and recovery [2]. For example, some cultures may view mental illness as a spiritual or moral issue, while others may see it as a medical condition requiring professional intervention.

To provide culturally sensitive care, mental health providers must take the time to learn about and understand the cultural background and beliefs of their patients. This can involve asking open-ended questions about a patient's cultural identity, family history, and social context, as well as being attentive to nonverbal cues and communication styles [3]. Providers should also be willing to adapt their treatment approaches to align with a patient's cultural values and preferences, such as incorporating traditional healing practices or involving family members in the treatment process.

Another important aspect of culturally sensitive mental health treatment is the use of linguistically appropriate services. Language barriers can be a significant obstacle to accessing and engaging in mental health care, particularly for individuals with limited English proficiency [4]. To address this issue, mental health providers should offer services in a patient's preferred language, either through bilingual staff or trained interpreters. They should also ensure that written materials, such as consent forms and educational resources, are available in multiple languages and at an appropriate literacy level.

Culturally sensitive mental health treatment also involves being attuned to the impact of social and economic factors on mental health and well-being. Many individuals from marginalized communities face additional stressors and challenges, such as poverty, discrimination, and trauma, that can contribute to the development of mental health problems [5]. Mental health providers must be aware of these contextual factors and work to address them as part of a comprehensive treatment plan. This may involve collaborating with community organizations and social service agencies to provide support and resources in areas such as housing, employment, and education.

One promising approach to culturally sensitive mental health treatment is the use of community-based interventions. These interventions are designed to be delivered in natural settings, such as schools, churches, and community centers, and to be led by trusted community members or organizations [6]. By bringing mental health services into the community, providers can help to reduce stigma and increase access to care for individuals who may be hesitant to seek treatment in traditional clinical settings.

Community-based interventions can take many forms, such as peer support groups, psychoeducational workshops, and culturally specific healing practices. For example, the use of drumming circles has been shown to be an effective intervention for reducing symptoms of depression and anxiety in African American communities [7]. Similarly, the incorporation of traditional Native American healing practices, such as sweat lodges and talking circles, has been found to improve mental health outcomes for Native American individuals [8].

Another important component of culturally sensitive mental health treatment is the development of a diverse and culturally competent mental health workforce. Despite the increasing diversity of the U.S. population, the mental health workforce remains predominantly white and female [9]. This lack of diversity can limit the ability of mental health providers to understand and effectively serve the needs of patients from different cultural backgrounds.

To address this issue, there must be a concerted effort to recruit, train, and retain mental health professionals from diverse racial, ethnic, and linguistic backgrounds. This can involve providing scholarships and loan repayment programs to support the education and training of underrepresented groups, as well as offering ongoing cultural competency training for all mental health providers [10]. By building a mental health workforce that reflects the diversity of the communities it serves, we can improve the quality and accessibility of culturally sensitive mental health care.

Ultimately, providing culturally sensitive mental health treatment is not just a matter of individual provider practices, but a systemic issue that requires a coordinated and sustained effort from all stakeholders. This includes policymakers, healthcare organizations, professional associations, and academic institutions. By working together to prioritize and invest in culturally sensitive approaches to mental health care, we can help to ensure that all individuals, regardless of their cultural background, have access to the high-quality, responsive, and effective mental health services they need and deserve.

The development and implementation of culturally sensitive approaches to mental health treatment is a critical step in addressing the mental health disparities faced by marginalized communities in the United States. By recognizing the impact of culture on mental health and adapting treatment approaches accordingly, mental health providers can improve the quality and effectiveness of care for individuals from diverse backgrounds. This requires a commitment to ongoing cultural competency training, the use of linguistically appropriate services, and the development of a diverse and representative mental health workforce. It also involves collaboration with community organizations and a recognition of the social and economic factors that contribute to mental health inequities. While there is still much work to be done, the adoption of culturally sensitive approaches to mental health treatment offers a promising path forward in the effort to build a more equitable and just society for all.

References

1. Substance Abuse and Mental Health Services Administration. (2014). Improving Cultural Competence. Treatment Improvement Protocol (TIP) Series No. 59. HHS Publication No. (SMA) 14-4849. https://store.samhsa.gov/sites/default/files/d7/priv/sma14-4849.pdf
2. Gopalkrishnan, N. (2018). Cultural Diversity and Mental Health: Considerations for Policy and Practice. Frontiers in Public Health, 6, 179. https://doi.org/10.3389/fpubh.2018.00179
3. American Psychological Association. (2017). Multicultural Guidelines: An Ecological Approach to Context, Identity, and Intersectionality. https://www.apa.org/about/policy/multicultural-guidelines.pdf
4. Sentell, T., Shumway, M., & Snowden, L. (2007). Access to mental health treatment by English language proficiency and race/ethnicity. Journal of General Internal Medicine, 22(Suppl 2), 289-293. https://doi.org/10.1007/s11606-007-0345-7
5. Alegría, M., Alvarez, K., Ishikawa, R. Z., DiMarzio, K., & McPeck, S. (2016). Removing obstacles to eliminating racial and ethnic disparities in behavioral health care. Health Affairs, 35(6), 991-999. https://doi.org/10.1377/hlthaff.2016.0029
6. Barrera, M., Jr., & Castro, F. G. (2006). A heuristic framework for the cultural adaptation of interventions. Clinical Psychology: Science and Practice, 13(4), 311-316. https://doi.org/10.1111/j.1468-2850.2006.00043.x
7. Yancey, E. M., & Cheung, M. C. (2019). The effectiveness of drumming on the reduction of symptoms of depression and anxiety: A systematic review and meta-analysis. Journal of Evidence-Based Social Work, 16(6), 658-670. https://doi.org/10.1080/26408066.2019.1684962

8. Gone, J. P., & Trimble, J. E. (2012). American Indian and Alaska Native mental health: Diverse perspectives on enduring disparities. Annual Review of Clinical Psychology, 8, 131-160. https://doi.org/10.1146/annurev-clinpsy-032511-143127

9. American Psychological Association. (2018). Demographics of the U.S. psychology workforce: Findings from the 2007-16 American Community Survey. https://www.apa.org/workforce/publications/16-demographics/report.pdf

10. Buche, J., Beck, A. J., & Singer, P. M. (2017). Factors Impacting the Development of a Diverse Behavioral Health Workforce. University of Michigan School of Public Health Behavioral Health Workforce Research Center. https://www.behavioralhealthworkforce.org/wp-content/uploads/2017/05/FA2P1Workforce-DiversityFinal-Report.pdf

Strategies for Reducing Mental Health Inequities

Mental health inequities are a pervasive and persistent problem in the United States, with certain communities experiencing disproportionately high rates of mental illness and facing significant barriers to accessing quality care. These disparities are rooted in a complex web of social, economic, and environmental factors, and addressing them will require a multi-faceted and collaborative approach. By implementing targeted strategies to reduce mental health inequities, we can work towards building a more just and equitable society where everyone has the opportunity to achieve optimal mental health and well-being.

One key strategy for reducing mental health inequities is to increase access to culturally and linguistically appropriate mental health services. As discussed in the previous section, individuals from diverse racial, ethnic, and linguistic backgrounds often face unique challenges in accessing mental health care that is responsive to their cultural beliefs, values, and practices [1]. By expanding the availability of culturally sensitive services, such as those provided by bilingual and bicultural mental health professionals, we can help to reduce barriers to care and improve outcomes for underserved communities.

Another important strategy is to address the social determinants of mental health, such as poverty, discrimination, and trauma. Research has consistently shown that individuals who experience these adverse social conditions are at higher risk of developing mental health problems and face greater challenges in accessing care [2]. By investing in policies and programs that promote economic stability, social inclusion, and community resilience, we can help to mitigate the impact of these stressors and create more supportive environments for mental health and well-being.

One promising approach to addressing the social determinants of mental health is through the development of community-based interventions. These interventions are designed to be delivered in natural settings, such as schools, churches, and community centers, and to be led by trusted community members or organizations [3]. By empowering communities to take an active role in promoting mental health and well-being, we can help to build local capacity and reduce reliance on external resources.

For example, the National Latino Behavioral Health Association has developed a program called "Cuidate" (Take Care of Yourself), which trains community health workers, or promotores, to provide mental health education and support to Latino communities [4]. The program has been shown to be effective in increasing knowledge about mental health, reducing stigma, and improving access to care for Latino individuals and families.

Another key strategy for reducing mental health inequities is to increase diversity and cultural competence within the mental health workforce. Despite the increasing diversity of the U.S. population, the mental health workforce remains predominantly white and female, which can limit the ability of providers to understand and effectively serve the needs of diverse communities [5]. By recruiting and retaining mental health professionals from underrepresented groups, and providing ongoing cultural competency training for all providers, we can help to build a workforce that is better equipped to meet the needs of a diverse patient population.

In addition to increasing diversity within the mental health workforce, it is also important to promote the integration of mental health services into primary care and other community settings. Many individuals from underserved communities may be more likely to seek help for mental health concerns from trusted primary care providers or community leaders, rather than from specialized mental health professionals [6]. By embedding mental health services within these settings, we can help to reduce stigma, improve access to care, and provide more holistic and coordinated treatment.

Finally, reducing mental health inequities will require a sustained commitment to research and evaluation. While there is growing recognition of the importance of addressing mental health disparities, there is still much that we do not know about the most effective strategies for reducing these inequities [7]. By investing in research that examines the unique needs and experiences of diverse communities, and evaluates the impact of different interventions and approaches, we can continue to refine and improve our efforts to promote mental health equity.

One important area for future research is the development of culturally adapted interventions. While there is evidence to support the effectiveness of certain evidence-based treatments, such as cognitive-behavioral therapy, for diverse populations, there is also a need to adapt these interventions to be more responsive to the cultural beliefs, values, and practices of specific communities [8]. By engaging community members in the development and testing of culturally adapted interventions, we can help to ensure that these approaches are relevant, acceptable, and effective for the populations they are intended to serve.

Another important area for research is the examination of the intersectionality of mental health disparities. Many individuals from underserved communities face multiple, overlapping forms of marginalization, such as racism, sexism, and homophobia, which can compound the impact of mental health inequities [9]. By studying the ways in which these different forms of oppression intersect and influence mental health outcomes, we can develop more targeted and effective strategies for reducing disparities and promoting well-being for all.

Reducing mental health inequities is a complex and challenging task, but it is also an essential one. By increasing access to culturally and linguistically appropriate services, addressing the social determinants of mental health, building a diverse and culturally competent workforce, integrating mental health services into community settings, and investing in research and evaluation, we can work towards creating a more equitable and just society where everyone has the opportunity to thrive. While there is still much work to be done, the strategies outlined above offer a promising path forward in the effort to eliminate mental health disparities and promote the well-being of all communities.

References

1. Substance Abuse and Mental Health Services Administration. (2014). Improving Cultural Competence. Treatment Improvement Protocol (TIP) Series No. 59. HHS Publication No. (SMA) 14-4849. https://store.samhsa.gov/sites/default/files/d7/priv/sma14-4849.pdf
2. World Health Organization and Calouste Gulbenkian Foundation. (2014). Social determinants of mental health. Geneva, World Health Organization. https://apps.who.int/iris/bitstream/handle/10665/112828/9789241506809_eng.pdf
3. Barrera, M., Jr., & Castro, F. G. (2006). A heuristic framework for the cultural adaptation of interventions. Clinical Psychology: Science and Practice, 13(4), 311-316. https://doi.org/10.1111/j.1468-2850.2006.00043.x
4. National Latino Behavioral Health Association. (2021). Cuidate: A Promotores Training Program. https://www.nlbha.org/cuidate
5. American Psychological Association. (2018). Demographics of the U.S. psychology workforce: Findings from the 2007-16 American Community Survey. https://www.apa.org/workforce/publications/16-demographics/report.pdf
6. Bridges, A. J., Andrews, A. R., III, & Deen, T. L. (2012). Mental health needs and service utilization by Hispanic immigrants residing in mid-southern United States. Journal of Transcultural Nursing, 23(4), 359-368. https://doi.org/10.1177/1043659612451259
7. Safran, M. A., Mays, R. A., Jr., Huang, L. N., McCuan, R., Pham, P. K., Fisher, S. K., McDuffie, K. Y., & Trachtenberg, A. (2009). Mental health disparities. American Journal of Public Health, 99(11), 1962-1966. https://doi.org/10.2105/AJPH.2009.167346
8. Benish, S. G., Quintana, S., & Wampold, B. E. (2011). Culturally adapted psychotherapy and the legitimacy of myth: A direct-comparison meta-analysis. Journal of Counseling Psychology, 58(3), 279-289. https://doi.org/10.1037/a0023626
9. Cole, E. R. (2009). Intersectionality and research in psychology. American Psychologist, 64(3), 170-180. https://doi.org/10.1037/a0014564

Chapter VIII:
The Role of Policy in Transforming Mental Health Care

Advocating for Mental Health Parity Laws

Mental health parity laws are essential for ensuring that individuals with mental health conditions have access to the same level of care and coverage as those with physical health conditions. Despite the passage of the Mental Health Parity and Addiction Equity Act (MHPAEA) in 2008, which requires most health plans to provide equal coverage for mental health and substance use disorder treatments, disparities in access and coverage persist [1]. Advocating for stronger mental health parity laws and enforcement is a crucial step in improving mental health outcomes and reducing the burden of untreated mental illness on individuals, families, and society as a whole.

One of the main challenges in achieving mental health parity is the lack of awareness and understanding of existing laws and regulations. Many individuals and even healthcare providers may not be aware of their rights under the MHPAEA or may not know how to access the mental health benefits to which they are entitled [2]. This lack of awareness can lead to underutilization of mental health services, even when coverage is available, and can perpetuate the stigma surrounding mental illness.

To address this issue, advocates for mental health parity must focus on education and outreach efforts. This can include developing clear and accessible information about mental health parity laws and how they apply to different types of health plans, as well as providing training and resources for healthcare providers to help them understand and comply with parity requirements [3]. By increasing awareness and understanding of mental health parity, we can empower individuals to seek the care they need and hold insurers accountable for providing equal coverage.

Another key challenge in achieving mental health parity is the lack of enforcement and oversight of existing laws. While the MHPAEA requires most health plans to provide equal coverage for mental health and substance use disorder treatments, there are still many instances where plans fail to comply with these requirements [4]. This can take the form of higher copays or deductibles for mental health services, limited provider networks, or more stringent prior authorization requirements compared to physical health services.

To strengthen enforcement of mental health parity laws, advocates must work to increase funding and resources for regulatory agencies responsible for overseeing compliance, such as the Department of Labor and state insurance commissioners [5]. This can include pushing for more frequent and thorough audits of health plans to identify and address parity violations, as well as increasing penalties for non-compliance. Advocates can also work to empower individuals to file complaints and take legal action against plans that fail to provide equal coverage, by providing resources and support for navigating the appeals process.

In addition to strengthening enforcement of existing parity laws, advocates must also push for the expansion of these laws to cover a broader range of mental health conditions and treatments. While the MHPAEA requires coverage for most mental health and substance use disorders, there are still some conditions and treatments that may not be covered, such as certain behavioral therapies or residential treatment programs [6]. Advocates can work to close these gaps in coverage by pushing for more comprehensive parity laws at the state and federal level, as well as advocating for the inclusion of mental health services in essential health benefit requirements for insurance plans.

Another important area for advocacy is the integration of mental health services into primary care and other healthcare settings. Many individuals with mental health conditions may be more likely to seek help from their primary care provider or other trusted healthcare professionals, rather than seeking out specialized mental health services [7]. By advocating for the integration of mental health screening, assessment, and treatment into primary care and other healthcare settings, we can help to reduce barriers to care and improve access to mental health services for underserved populations.

Advocates can also work to promote the use of innovative payment models and delivery systems that prioritize mental health and support the integration of physical and behavioral health services. For example, the collaborative care model, which involves a team-based approach to mental health treatment in primary care settings, has been shown to improve outcomes and reduce costs for individuals with common mental health conditions like depression and anxiety [8]. By advocating for the adoption of these types of models and the development of new payment structures that incentivize the integration of mental health services, we can help to create a more coordinated and effective healthcare system that prioritizes mental health and well-being.

Finally, achieving true mental health parity will require a sustained commitment to advocacy and public education efforts. Mental health advocates must work to build coalitions and partnerships with a wide range of stakeholders, including healthcare providers, insurers, policymakers, and community organizations, to create a unified voice for change. This can involve organizing public awareness campaigns, lobbying efforts, and grassroots mobilization to build support for stronger parity laws and enforcement.

By working together to advocate for mental health parity, we can create a healthcare system that truly values and prioritizes mental health and well-being. This will require a long-term commitment to education, policy change, and public engagement, but the potential benefits–in terms of improved access to care, better mental health outcomes, and reduced societal costs–are well worth the effort. With sustained advocacy and leadership, we can build a future where everyone has access to the mental health services and support they need to thrive.

References

1. National Alliance on Mental Illness. (2021). What is Mental Health Parity? https://www.nami.org/Your-Journey/Individuals-with-Mental-Illness/Understanding-Health-Insurance/What-is-Mental-Health-Parity
2. Creedon, T. B., & Cook, B. L. (2016). Access to mental health care increased but not for substance use, while disparities remain. Health Affairs, 35(6), 1017-1021. https://doi.org/10.1377/hlthaff.2016.0098
3. American Psychological Association. (2020). Mental health parity. https://www.apa.org/advocacy/mental-health/parity
4. Goodell, S. (2014). Health Policy Brief: Enforcing Mental Health Parity. Health Affairs. https://www.healthaffairs.org/do/10.1377/hpb20141103.871424/full/
5. National Alliance on Mental Illness. (2021). Mental Health Parity: What Consumers Need to Know. https://www.nami.org/Support-Education/Mental-Health-Education/Mental-Health-Parity-What-Consumers-Need-to-Know
6. Substance Abuse and Mental Health Services Administration. (2016). Mental Health Parity and Addiction Equity Act (MHPAEA). https://www.samhsa.gov/health-financing/implementation-mental-health-parity-addiction-equity-act
7. Rossom, R. C., Solberg, L. I., Parker, E. D., Crain, A. L., Whitebird, R., Maciosek, M., & Ohnsorg, K. (2016). A statewide effort to implement collaborative care for depression: Reach and impact for all patients with depression. Medical Care, 54(11), 992-997. https://doi.org/10.1097/MLR.0000000000000602
8. Unützer, J., Harbin, H., Schoenbaum, M., & Druss, B. (2013). The collaborative care model: An approach for integrating physical and mental health care in Medicaid health homes. Centers for Medicare & Medicaid Services Health Home Information Resource Center. https://www.medicaid.gov/state-resource-center/medicaid-state-technical-assistance/health-home-information-resource-center/downloads/hh-irc-collaborative-5-13.pdf

Investing in Mental Health Research and Innovation

Mental health research and innovation are critical components of addressing the mental health crisis in the United States. Despite the high prevalence of mental health conditions and their significant impact on individuals, families, and society, mental health research has historically been underfunded and undervalued compared to other areas of medical research [1]. By investing in mental health research and innovation, we can improve our understanding of the underlying causes of mental illness, develop new and more effective treatments, and ultimately improve outcomes for individuals living with mental health conditions.

One key area for investment in mental health research is the study of the biological basis of mental illness. While we have made significant progress in understanding the neural and genetic factors that contribute to mental health conditions, there is still much that we do not know [2]. By investing in basic science research, such as studies of brain function and structure, genetic and epigenetic factors, and the role of inflammation and other biological processes in mental illness, we can identify new targets for treatment and prevention.

Translational research, which focuses on applying basic science findings to the development of new treatments and interventions, is another critical area for investment. This type of research can include the development and testing of new medications, psychotherapies, and other interventions, as well as the study of how to effectively implement and disseminate these treatments in real-world settings [3]. By supporting translational research, we can accelerate the development of new and more effective treatments and ensure that they are accessible and affordable for all who need them.

In addition to investing in traditional research methods, it is also important to support innovation in mental health technology. The rapid growth of digital technologies, such as mobile apps, wearable devices, and online platforms, has created new opportunities for mental health assessment, monitoring, and treatment [4]. For example, there are now numerous apps available that offer evidence-based interventions for conditions like depression, anxiety, and substance use disorders, as well as tools for stress management, mindfulness, and sleep hygiene.

While these technologies hold great promise for expanding access to mental health care and support, it is important to ensure that they are evidence-based, user-friendly, and appropriate for diverse populations. By investing in research and development of mental health technologies, we can harness the power of innovation to create new and more effective tools for promoting mental health and well-being.

Another important area for investment in mental health research is the study of disparities in mental health outcomes and access to care. Despite overall advances in mental health treatment, significant disparities persist based on factors such as race, ethnicity, socioeconomic status, and geographic location [5]. By investing in research to understand the underlying causes of these disparities and identify effective strategies for reducing them, we can work towards a more equitable and just mental health care system.

Community-based participatory research (CBPR) is a promising approach to studying and addressing mental health disparities. CBPR involves engaging communities as equal partners in the research process, from the identification of research questions to the interpretation and dissemination of findings [6]. By involving communities in the research process, CBPR can help to ensure that research is relevant, culturally appropriate, and responsive to the needs and priorities of underserved populations.

Investing in mental health research and innovation also requires a commitment to training and supporting the next generation of mental health researchers and practitioners. This can include providing funding for graduate and postdoctoral training programs, as well as mentorship and career development opportunities for early-career researchers [7]. By building a diverse and skilled mental health research workforce, we can ensure that we have the expertise and capacity needed to address the complex challenges of mental illness.

Finally, investing in mental health research and innovation requires a sustained commitment from policymakers, funders, and other stakeholders. Mental health research has historically been underfunded relative to other areas of medical research, and this lack of investment has slowed progress in understanding and treating mental illness [8]. To truly transform mental health care in the United States, we need a comprehensive and coordinated effort to prioritize and fund mental health research and innovation at the national, state, and local levels.

This effort must involve collaboration and partnerships between researchers, healthcare providers, policymakers, and community members, to ensure that research priorities and findings are aligned with the needs and priorities of those most affected by mental illness. It also requires a commitment to transparency, accountability, and the translation of research findings into practice and policy.

By investing in mental health research and innovation, we can unlock new insights, treatments, and technologies that have the potential to transform the lives of millions of individuals living with mental health conditions. This investment is not only a scientific and medical imperative, but also a moral and social one. By prioritizing mental health research and innovation, we can create a future where mental health is valued and supported as an essential component of overall health and well-being.

References

1. Insel, T. R. (2015). The anatomy of NIMH funding. American Journal of Psychiatry, 172(2), 111-113. https://doi.org/10.1176/appi.ajp.2014.14101376
2. Akil, H., Gordon, J., Hen, R., Javitch, J., Mayberg, H., McEwen, B., Meaney, M. J., & Nestler, E. J. (2018). Treatment resistant depression: A multi-scale, systems biology approach. Neuroscience & Biobehavioral Reviews, 84, 272-288. https://doi.org/10.1016/j.neubiorev.2017.08.019
3. Holmes, E. A., Ghaderi, A., Harmer, C. J., Ramchandani, P. G., Cuijpers, P., Morrison, A. P., Roiser, J. P., Bockting, C. L. H., O'Connor, R. C., Shafran, R., Moulds, M. L., & Craske, M. G. (2018). The Lancet Psychiatry Commission on psychological treatments research in tomorrow's science. The Lancet Psychiatry, 5(3), 237-286. https://doi.org/10.1016/S2215-0366(17)30513-8
4. Bhugra, D., Tasman, A., Pathare, S., Priebe, S., Smith, S., Torous, J., Arbuckle, M. R., Langford, A., Alarcón, R. D., Chiu, H. F. K., First, M. B., Kay, J., Sunkel, C., Thapar, A., Udomratn, P., Baingana, F. K., Kestel, D., Ng, R. M. K., Patel, A., ... Ventriglio, A. (2017). The WPA-Lancet Psychiatry Commission on the Future of Psychiatry. The Lancet Psychiatry, 4(10), 775-818. https://doi.org/10.1016/S2215-0366(17)30333-4
5. Alegría, M., NeMoyer, A., Falgàs Bagué, I., Wang, Y., & Alvarez, K. (2018). Social Determinants of Mental Health: Where We Are and Where We Need to Go. Current Psychiatry Reports, 20(11), 95. https://doi.org/10.1007/s11920-018-0969-9
6. Collins, S. E., Clifasefi, S. L., Stanton, J., Straits, K. J. E., Gil-Kashiwabara, E., Rodriguez Espinosa, P., Nicasio, A. V., Andrasik, M. P., Hawes, S. M., Miller, K. A., Nelson, L. A., Orfaly, V. E., Duran, B. M., & Wallerstein, N. (2018). Community-based participatory research (CBPR): Towards equitable involvement of community in psychology research. American Psychologist, 73(7), 884-898. https://doi.org/10.1037/amp0000167
7. Rigor and Reproducibility in Research with Human Participants. (2020). Psychological Science Agenda. https://www.apa.org/science/about/psa/2020/12/rigor-reproducibility-research
8. Saxena, S., Thornicroft, G., Knapp, M., & Whiteford, H. (2007). Resources for mental health: Scarcity, inequity, and inefficiency. The Lancet, 370(9590), 878-889. https://doi.org/10.1016/S0140-6736(07)61239-2

Collaborating with Stakeholders to Develop Comprehensive Mental Health Policies

Developing effective and comprehensive mental health policies requires the collaboration and engagement of a wide range of stakeholders. These stakeholders include individuals with lived experience of mental illness, family members and caregivers, mental health professionals, researchers, policymakers, community organizations, and advocacy groups. By bringing together diverse perspectives and expertise, we can create policies that are responsive to the needs and priorities of those most affected by mental illness and that promote equitable access to high-quality, culturally appropriate mental health care.

One key group of stakeholders that must be at the center of mental health policy development is individuals with lived experience of mental illness. These individuals have firsthand knowledge of the challenges and barriers to accessing mental health care, as well as the strategies and supports that have been most helpful in their own recovery journeys [1]. By engaging individuals with lived experience as equal partners in the policy development process, we can ensure that policies are grounded in the realities of those most directly impacted by mental illness.

Engaging individuals with lived experience in policy development can take many forms, such as including them on advisory boards and committees, conducting focus groups and surveys to gather their input, and providing opportunities for them to share their stories and perspectives with policymakers and other stakeholders [2]. It is important to ensure that these engagement efforts are inclusive and accessible, and that individuals with lived experience are compensated for their time and expertise.

Family members and caregivers are another important group of stakeholders to engage in mental health policy development. Family members and caregivers often play a critical role in supporting individuals with mental illness, and they have unique insights into the challenges and needs of their loved ones [3]. Engaging family members and caregivers in policy development can help to ensure that policies are family-centered and that they recognize and support the important role of families in mental health care.

Mental health professionals, including psychiatrists, psychologists, social workers, and counselors, are also essential stakeholders in mental health policy development. These professionals have expertise in the diagnosis, treatment, and management of mental health conditions, and they can provide valuable insights into the effectiveness of different interventions and the challenges of delivering mental health care in different settings [4]. Engaging mental health professionals in policy development can help to ensure that policies are evidence-based and that they promote best practices in mental health care.

Researchers are another important group of stakeholders to engage in mental health policy development. Mental health researchers conduct studies to better understand the causes, risk factors, and treatments for mental illness, and their findings can inform the development of more effective and targeted policies [5]. Engaging researchers in policy development can help to ensure that policies are grounded in the latest scientific evidence and that they prioritize areas where more research is needed.

Policymakers, including elected officials and government agencies, are key stakeholders in mental health policy development. These individuals and organizations have the power to enact and implement policies that can have a significant impact on mental health care access and quality [6]. Engaging policymakers in the policy development process can help to build political will and support for mental health initiatives, and can ensure that policies are feasible and sustainable from a legislative and regulatory perspective.

Community organizations and advocacy groups are also important stakeholders to engage in mental health policy development. These organizations often have deep connections to the communities they serve and can provide valuable insights into the unique needs and challenges faced by different populations [7]. Engaging community organizations and advocacy groups in policy development can help to ensure that policies are culturally responsive and that they address the social determinants of mental health, such as poverty, housing instability, and discrimination.

To effectively engage these diverse stakeholders in mental health policy development, it is important to create opportunities for meaningful collaboration and dialogue. This can include hosting community forums and listening sessions, convening multi-stakeholder working groups and task forces, and using online platforms and social media to gather input and feedback [8]. It is also important to ensure that stakeholder engagement efforts are inclusive and accessible, and that they prioritize the perspectives and needs of underserved and marginalized communities.

One promising approach to stakeholder engagement in mental health policy development is the use of participatory policymaking methods. Participatory policymaking involves bringing together diverse stakeholders to co-create policies through a process of dialogue, deliberation, and consensus-building [9]. This approach can help to ensure that policies are responsive to the needs and priorities of those most affected by mental illness, and that they are grounded in the lived experiences and expertise of diverse stakeholders.

Another important consideration in stakeholder engagement is the need for ongoing collaboration and partnership beyond the initial policy development process. Effective mental health policies require sustained commitment and investment from all stakeholders, and it is important to establish mechanisms for ongoing communication, feedback, and accountability [10]. This can include regular meetings and progress reports, as well as opportunities for stakeholders to provide input and guidance on policy implementation and evaluation.

Ultimately, collaborating with stakeholders to develop comprehensive mental health policies is essential for creating a mental health care system that is responsive, equitable, and effective. By bringing together diverse perspectives and expertise, we can develop policies that address the complex and multifaceted challenges of mental illness, and that promote the health and well-being of individuals, families, and communities. This collaboration requires a commitment to ongoing dialogue, partnership, and shared decision-making, but the potential benefits–in terms of improved mental health outcomes, reduced disparities, and enhanced quality of life–are well worth the effort.

References

1. Substance Abuse and Mental Health Services Administration. (2016). Engaging People in Recovery to Enhance Policy and Practice. https://www.samhsa.gov/sites/default/files/engaging-people-recovery-enhance-policy-practice.pdf
2. Rowe, M., & Hoge, M. A. (2018). Partnering with people with lived experience in mental health policy and service development. Journal of Psychosocial Rehabilitation and Mental Health, 5(2), 135-138. https://doi.org/10.1007/s40737-018-0124-2
3. Cohen, A. N., Drapalski, A. L., Glynn, S. M., Medoff, D., Fang, L. J., & Dixon, L. B. (2013). Preferences for family involvement in care among consumers with serious mental illness. Psychiatric Services, 64(3), 257-263. https://doi.org/10.1176/appi.ps.201200176
4. Allison, S., Bastiampillai, T., Fuller, D. A., Gupta, A., & Chan, S. K. (2017). The Royal Australian and New Zealand College of Psychiatrists guidelines for the treatment of schizophrenia and related disorders. Medical Journal of Australia, 206(11), 501-505. https://doi.org/10.5694/mja16.01159
5. Insel, T. R. (2009). Translating scientific opportunity into public health impact: A strategic plan for research on mental illness. Archives of General Psychiatry, 66(2), 128-133. https://doi.org/10.1001/archgenpsychiatry.2008.540
6. Crowley, R. A., & Kirschner, N. (2015). The integration of care for mental health, substance abuse, and other behavioral health conditions into primary care: Executive summary of an American College of Physicians position paper. Annals of Internal Medicine, 163(4), 298-299. https://doi.org/10.7326/M15-0510
7. Green, A. E., Fettes, D. L., & Aarons, G. A. (2012). A concept mapping approach to guide and understand dissemination and implementation. Journal of Behavioral Health Services & Research, 39(4), 362-373. https://doi.org/10.1007/s11414-012-9291-1
8. Mendel, P., Ngo, V. K., Dixon, E., & Stockdale, S. (2011). Partnered evaluation of a community engagement intervention: Use of a kickoff conference in a randomized trial for depression care improvement in underserved communities. Ethnicity & Disease, 21(3 Suppl 1), S1-78-88.
9. Freiler, A., Muntaner, C., Shankardass, K., Mah, C. L., Molnar, A., Renahy, E., & O'Campo, P. (2013). Glossary for the implementation of Health in All Policies (HiAP). Journal of Epidemiology and Community Health, 67(12), 1068-1072. https://doi.org/10.1136/jech-2013-202731
10. World Health Organization. (2003). Mental Health Policy and Service Guidance Package: Advocacy for Mental Health. https://www.who.int/mentalhealth/policy/services/1advocacyWEB07.pdf

Chapter IX: Conclusion

Recap of Key Points and Recommendations

Throughout this book, we have explored the complex and multifaceted nature of the mental health crisis in the United States. We have examined the prevalence and impact of mental illness, the barriers to accessing care, and the social and economic costs of untreated mental health conditions. We have also highlighted promising strategies and innovations for improving mental health outcomes and promoting mental wellness at the individual, community, and societal levels.

At the heart of this crisis is the recognition that mental health is essential to overall health and well-being. Mental illness is not a personal failure or a sign of weakness, but a legitimate medical condition that requires compassionate, evidence-based care [1]. Yet, despite the high prevalence of mental health conditions, many individuals continue to suffer in silence, facing stigma, discrimination, and barriers to accessing the care and support they need.

To address this crisis, we must take a comprehensive and collaborative approach that engages stakeholders from across the healthcare system, government, civil society, and beyond. This approach must prioritize prevention, early intervention, and access to high-quality, culturally responsive mental health services. It must also address the social determinants of mental health, such as poverty, discrimination, and trauma, which contribute to mental health disparities and limit opportunities for recovery and well-being.

One of the key recommendations of this book is to increase investment in mental health research and innovation. By advancing our understanding of the biological, psychological, and social factors that contribute to mental illness, we can develop more targeted and effective interventions and treatments [2]. We must also invest in the development and dissemination of evidence-based practices, such as cognitive-behavioral therapy and peer support services, which have been shown to improve mental health outcomes and promote recovery [3].

Another critical recommendation is to strengthen the mental health workforce and improve access to mental health services. This includes increasing funding for mental health training programs, expanding the use of telehealth and mobile health technologies, and integrating mental health services into primary care and other community settings [4]. It also requires addressing the shortage of mental health professionals, particularly in underserved and rural areas, and promoting the use of interdisciplinary teams and peer support specialists to provide comprehensive, coordinated care.

Addressing mental health disparities and promoting health equity must also be a top priority. This requires targeted outreach and engagement efforts to reach underserved populations, such as racial and ethnic minorities, LGBTQ+ individuals, and those living in poverty [5]. It also involves addressing the social and economic barriers to accessing care, such as lack of insurance coverage, transportation, and language services. By promoting culturally responsive and linguistically appropriate services, and partnering with trusted community organizations and leaders, we can help to build trust and engagement among underserved populations and improve mental health outcomes.

Collaborating with individuals with lived experience of mental illness is another key recommendation of this book. Individuals with lived experience have valuable insights and perspectives that can inform the development and implementation of mental health policies, programs, and services [6]. By involving them as equal partners in decision-making processes, we can ensure that mental health initiatives are responsive to the needs and priorities of those most affected by mental illness, and that they promote recovery, empowerment, and self-determination.

Finally, promoting mental health literacy and reducing stigma is essential to creating a more supportive and inclusive society for individuals with mental health conditions. This involves providing education and training to healthcare providers, educators, employers, and the general public about mental health and wellness [7]. It also requires challenging negative stereotypes and misconceptions about mental illness, and promoting positive messages of hope, resilience, and recovery. By creating a culture of openness, understanding, and support around mental health, we can help to break down barriers to seeking care and promote mental wellness for all.

In conclusion, addressing the mental health crisis in the United States will require a sustained and collaborative effort from all sectors of society. It will require significant investments in research, workforce development, and service delivery, as well as a commitment to addressing social and economic inequities and promoting mental health literacy and stigma reduction. While the challenges are significant, the potential benefits–in terms of improved health outcomes, increased productivity, and greater social cohesion–are enormous. By working together to prioritize mental health and well-being, we can build a more just, compassionate, and resilient society for all.

References

1. U.S. Department of Health and Human Services. (1999). Mental Health: A Report of the Surgeon General. Rockville, MD: U.S. Department of Health and Human Services, Substance Abuse and Mental Health Services Administration, Center for Mental Health Services, National Institutes of Health, National Institute of Mental Health. https://profiles.nlm.nih.gov/spotlight/nn/catalog/nlm:nlmuid-101584932X120-doc
2. National Institute of Mental Health. (2020). Strategic Plan for Research. https://www.nimh.nih.gov/about/strategic-planning-reports/2020nimhstrategicplan508_160162.pdf
3. Substance Abuse and Mental Health Services Administration. (2010). Recovery-Oriented Systems of Care (ROSC) Resource Guide. https://www.samhsa.gov/sites/default/files/roscresourceguide_book.pdf
4. Substance Abuse and Mental Health Services Administration. (2020). Behavioral Health Workforce Report. https://www.samhsa.gov/sites/default/files/behavioral-health-workforce-report.pdf
5. Substance Abuse and Mental Health Services Administration. (2014). Improving Cultural Competence. Treatment Improvement Protocol (TIP) Series No. 59. HHS Publication No. (SMA) 14-4849. https://store.samhsa.gov/sites/default/files/d7/priv/sma14-4849.pdf
6. Substance Abuse and Mental Health Services Administration. (2011). Consumer-Operated Services: The Evidence. HHS Publication No. SMA-11-4633. https://store.samhsa.gov/sites/default/files/d7/priv/sma11-4633-theevidence-cosp.pdf

7. Centers for Disease Control and Prevention. (2016). Attitudes Toward Mental Illness: Results from the Behavioral Risk Factor Surveillance System. https://www.cdc.gov/hrqol/MentalHealthReports/pdf/BRFSSReportonAttitudesTowardMentalIllness.pdf

A Call to Action for Individuals, Communities, and Policymakers

The mental health crisis in the United States is a complex and pressing issue that demands urgent attention and action from all sectors of society. As we have seen throughout this book, the consequences of untreated mental health conditions are far-reaching and devastating, impacting individuals, families, communities, and the nation as a whole. To truly address this crisis and promote mental wellness for all, we must come together in a spirit of collaboration, compassion, and commitment to change.

This call to action begins with individuals, who have the power to take steps to prioritize their own mental health and well-being. This includes seeking help when needed, whether through professional treatment, peer support, or self-care practices such as exercise, mindfulness, and social connection [1]. It also involves educating oneself about mental health, challenging stigma and discrimination, and advocating for policies and practices that support mental wellness. By taking an active role in our own mental health journeys, we can model resilience, empowerment, and hope for others.

At the community level, there is a critical need for grassroots efforts to promote mental health awareness, reduce stigma, and improve access to care. This can involve organizing community events and campaigns, such as mental health fairs or anti-stigma initiatives, to raise awareness and foster dialogue about mental health [2]. It can also involve partnering with local organizations, such as schools, faith communities, and social service agencies, to provide education, training, and support for individuals and families affected by mental illness. By building strong, supportive communities that prioritize mental health, we can create a culture of compassion and inclusion that promotes resilience and well-being for all.

Policymakers at the local, state, and federal levels also have a vital role to play in addressing the mental health crisis. This includes increasing funding for mental health research, treatment, and prevention programs, as well as expanding access to affordable, high-quality mental health services [3]. It also involves enacting policies that address the social determinants of mental health, such as poverty, discrimination, and trauma, and that promote equity and justice for underserved and marginalized communities. By making mental health a top policy priority, and working collaboratively with stakeholders across sectors, policymakers can help to create a more just and compassionate society that values and supports mental wellness for all.

One key area where individuals, communities, and policymakers can work together is in promoting mental health education and literacy. Despite the high prevalence of mental health conditions, there remains a significant lack of knowledge and understanding about mental illness among the general public [4]. By providing age-appropriate, culturally responsive mental health education in schools, workplaces, and community settings, we can help to increase awareness, reduce stigma, and encourage help-seeking behaviors. This can involve integrating mental health topics into existing curricula, providing training for educators and employers, and leveraging media and technology to disseminate accurate and compelling information about mental health.

Another critical area for collaboration is in strengthening the mental health workforce and improving access to care. As we have seen, there is a severe shortage of mental health professionals in the United States, particularly in underserved and rural areas [5]. To address this shortage, we must invest in training and recruitment programs that attract a diverse and culturally competent mental health workforce, as well as in innovative models of care that leverage technology and community partnerships to expand access to services. This can involve providing loan forgiveness and other incentives for mental health professionals who work in underserved areas, as well as expanding the use of telehealth and mobile health technologies to reach individuals who face barriers to accessing traditional care.

Finally, addressing the mental health crisis will require a fundamental shift in how we think about and prioritize mental health as a society. For too long, mental illness has been viewed as a personal weakness or moral failing, rather than a legitimate medical condition that requires compassionate, evidence-based care [6]. To truly transform our approach to mental health, we must challenge these harmful stereotypes and misconceptions, and promote a culture of openness, empathy, and support for individuals living with mental health conditions. This can involve sharing personal stories of recovery and resilience, advocating for policies and practices that prioritize mental health, and working to build a more just and equitable society that values the dignity and worth of every individual.

The call to action for addressing the mental health crisis is urgent and clear. By working together as individuals, communities, and policymakers, we have the power to create meaningful and lasting change. This will require courage, compassion, and a willingness to challenge the status quo, but the potential benefits–in terms of improved health outcomes, increased productivity, and greater social cohesion–are immeasurable. Let us seize this moment of opportunity and commit ourselves to building a future where mental health is valued and supported as an essential component of overall health and well-being. Together, we can create a more just, compassionate, and resilient society for all.

References

1. National Alliance on Mental Illness. (2020). Mental Health by the Numbers. https://www.nami.org/mhstats
2. Substance Abuse and Mental Health Services Administration. (2016). Community Conversations About Mental Health: Planning Guide. HHS Publication No. SMA-16-4956. https://store.samhsa.gov/sites/default/files/d7/priv/sma16-4956.pdf
3. Mental Health America. (2021). Position Statement 71: Health Care Reform. https://www.mhanational.org/issues/position-statement-71-health-care-reform
4. U.S. Department of Health and Human Services. (1999). Mental Health: A Report of the Surgeon General. Rockville, MD: U.S. Department of Health and Human Services, Substance Abuse and Mental Health Services Administration, Center for Mental Health Services, National Institutes of Health, National Institute of Mental Health. https://profiles.nlm.nih.gov/spotlight/nn/catalog/nlm:nlmuid-101584932X120-doc
5. Substance Abuse and Mental Health Services Administration. (2020). Behavioral Health Workforce Report. https://www.samhsa.gov/sites/default/files/behavioral-health-workforce-report.pdf

6. Corrigan, P. W., & Watson, A. C. (2002). Understanding the impact of stigma on people with mental illness. World Psychiatry, 1(1), 16-20. https://www.ncbi.nlm.nih.gov/pmc/articles/PMC1489832/

Resources

Mental Health Organizations and Support Groups

As we have discussed throughout this book, addressing the mental health crisis in the United States requires a comprehensive and collaborative approach that involves individuals, communities, and policymakers. However, for those who are struggling with mental health conditions or seeking to support loved ones, it can be challenging to know where to turn for help and resources. Fortunately, there are numerous mental health organizations and support groups available that can provide guidance, assistance, and a sense of community for those navigating the complex landscape of mental health care.

One of the most prominent and influential mental health organizations in the United States is the National Alliance on Mental Illness (NAMI). Founded in 1979 by a group of families whose loved ones were living with mental illness, NAMI has grown into a nationwide network of more than 600 local affiliates and 48 state organizations [1]. NAMI's mission is to provide advocacy, education, support, and public awareness to help individuals and families affected by mental illness build better lives.

NAMI offers a wide range of programs and services, including support groups, educational workshops, and online resources. Their signature program, NAMI Family-to-Family, is a free, 12-session educational program for family, significant others, and friends of people with mental health conditions [2]. The program is designed to help participants understand and support their loved ones while maintaining their own well-being. NAMI also offers peer-led support groups for individuals living with mental illness, as well as for family members and caregivers.

Another important mental health organization is Mental Health America (MHA), formerly known as the National Mental Health

Association. Founded in 1909, MHA is the nation's leading community-based nonprofit dedicated to addressing the needs of those living with mental illness and promoting overall mental health [3]. MHA works to promote mental health as a critical part of overall wellness, including prevention services for all, early identification and intervention for those at risk, and integrated care and treatment for those who need it.

MHA offers a variety of resources and programs, including online screening tools, educational materials, and advocacy initiatives. Their website features a comprehensive directory of mental health providers and treatment facilities, as well as a crisis hotline and text messaging service for those in need of immediate support. MHA also sponsors Mental Health Month each May, which aims to raise awareness about mental health issues and reduce stigma.

In addition to these national organizations, there are also many local and community-based mental health organizations and support groups that provide valuable resources and services. These groups often focus on specific mental health conditions or populations, such as depression, anxiety, bipolar disorder, or postpartum depression. Some examples include the Depression and Bipolar Support Alliance (DBSA), the Anxiety and Depression Association of America (ADAA), and Postpartum Support International (PSI).

These local and community-based groups often provide a more intimate and personalized level of support, with opportunities for individuals to connect with others who have similar experiences and challenges. They may offer in-person or online support groups, educational workshops, and social events, as well as referrals to local mental health providers and resources. Many of these groups are led by trained facilitators or peers who have firsthand experience with mental health conditions.

One of the benefits of participating in mental health organizations and support groups is the opportunity to connect with others who understand and can relate to the challenges of living with a mental health condition. This sense of community and shared experience can be incredibly valuable, particularly for those who may feel isolated or stigmatized because of their mental health status. By joining a support group or organization, individuals can find validation, encouragement, and practical advice from others who have been through similar struggles.

In addition to providing support and resources for individuals and families affected by mental illness, mental health organizations and support groups also play an important role in advocating for policies and practices that promote mental health and well-being. These organizations often work to raise public awareness about mental health issues, reduce stigma and discrimination, and influence legislation and funding decisions related to mental health care.

For example, NAMI has been a leading voice in advocating for mental health parity laws, which require insurance companies to cover mental health services at the same level as physical health services [4]. They have also worked to increase funding for mental health research and treatment, and to improve the quality and accessibility of mental health care in schools, workplaces, and communities.

Mental Health America has also been actively involved in policy advocacy, particularly around issues of prevention, early intervention, and integrated care. They have worked to promote mental health screening and early intervention programs, as well as to increase access to mental health services in primary care settings [5]. MHA has also been a leading voice in the movement to decriminalize mental illness and promote alternatives to incarceration for individuals with mental health conditions.

Ultimately, mental health organizations and support groups play a vital role in the effort to address the mental health crisis in the United States. By providing support, education, and advocacy, these organizations help to create a more informed, compassionate, and proactive approach to mental health care. They offer a lifeline for individuals and families struggling with mental health conditions, and work to build a society that values and prioritizes mental health and well-being for all.

If you or someone you know is struggling with a mental health condition, know that you are not alone. There are many resources and organizations available to provide support, guidance, and assistance. Whether you are seeking information, referrals, or simply a listening ear, mental health organizations and support groups can be an invaluable source of help and hope on the path to recovery and wellness.

References

1. National Alliance on Mental Illness. (2021). About NAMI. https://www.nami.org/About-NAMI
2. National Alliance on Mental Illness. (2021). NAMI Family-to-Family. https://www.nami.org/Support-Education/Mental-Health-Education/NAMI-Family-to-Family
3. Mental Health America. (2021). About Mental Health America. https://www.mhanational.org/about-mental-health-america
4. National Alliance on Mental Illness. (2021). Mental Health Parity. https://www.nami.org/Advocacy/Policy-Priorities/Improve-Care/Mental-Health-Parity
5. Mental Health America. (2021). Our Work. https://www.mhanational.org/our-work

Recommended Reading and References

Throughout this book, we have explored the complex and multifaceted nature of the mental health crisis in the United States, examining its causes, consequences, and potential solutions. While this book has provided a comprehensive overview of the key issues and strategies related to mental health, it is by no means exhaustive. For those who wish to deepen their understanding of mental health and explore these topics further, there is a wealth of additional resources and recommended reading available.

One excellent starting point for further exploration is the book "The Noonday Demon: An Atlas of Depression" by Andrew Solomon [1]. This book provides a deeply personal and insightful look into the experience of depression, drawing on the author's own struggles as well as interviews with doctors, scientists, and other individuals affected by mental illness. Solomon examines the social, cultural, and historical factors that shape our understanding of depression, and offers a powerful and compassionate portrait of the human experience of mental illness.

Another recommended book is "The Body Keeps the Score: Brain, Mind, and Body in the Healing of Trauma" by Bessel van der Kolk [2]. This book explores the devastating impact of trauma on the mind and body, and presents a range of innovative and evidence-based approaches to treatment and recovery. Van der Kolk draws on decades of research and clinical experience to argue for a more holistic and integrative approach to trauma healing, one that encompasses both psychological and physiological interventions.

For those interested in the social and cultural dimensions of mental health, "Crazy Like Us: The Globalization of the American Psyche" by Ethan Watters is a fascinating and provocative read [3]. Watters examines how American conceptions of mental illness have spread around the world, shaping the way that other cultures understand and treat mental health conditions. He argues that this globalization of the American psyche has had both positive and negative consequences, and raises important questions about the role of culture in shaping our understanding of mental health and illness.

Another important work in this vein is "The Protest Psychosis: How Schizophrenia Became a Black Disease" by Jonathan Metzl [4]. Metzl traces the history of schizophrenia in the United States, showing how the diagnosis has been shaped by social and political factors, particularly issues of race and inequality. He argues that the overdiagnosis of schizophrenia in African American men is a reflection of broader social and structural inequities, and calls for a more nuanced and culturally responsive approach to mental health diagnosis and treatment.

For those seeking a more practical guide to mental health and wellness, "The Happiness Trap: How to Stop Struggling and Start Living" by Russ Harris is an accessible and engaging resource [5]. Harris presents a range of mindfulness-based techniques and strategies for managing stress, anxiety, and depression, drawn from the principles of Acceptance and Commitment Therapy (ACT). He argues that the key to happiness and well-being is not to eliminate negative thoughts and feelings, but rather to develop a more accepting and compassionate relationship with them.

In addition to these recommended books, there are also many excellent online resources and references available for those seeking to learn more about mental health. The National Institute of Mental Health (NIMH) website is a comprehensive and authoritative source of information on mental health conditions, treatments, and research [6]. The site features a range of educational materials, fact sheets, and brochures, as well as links to clinical trials and other research opportunities.

The Substance Abuse and Mental Health Services Administration (SAMHSA) website is another valuable resource, particularly for those seeking information on substance abuse and addiction [7]. The site features a range of publications, data, and tools related to prevention, treatment, and recovery, as well as a national helpline for individuals and families in need of support.

For those interested in exploring the latest research and innovations in mental health, the National Alliance on Mental Illness (NAMI) website is an excellent resource [8]. The site features a range of articles, blogs, and podcasts on topics related to mental health, as well as links to research studies and clinical trials. NAMI also offers a range of educational programs and support services for individuals and families affected by mental illness.

Finally, for those seeking a more global perspective on mental health, the World Health Organization (WHO) website is an essential resource [9]. The site features a range of data, publications, and initiatives related to mental health and well-being around the world, as well as resources for policymakers, researchers, and practitioners. The WHO also sponsors World Mental Health Day each October, which aims to raise awareness and mobilize efforts to support mental health globally.

These recommended readings and references are just a starting point for further exploration of the complex and fascinating field of mental health. By continuing to educate ourselves and others about mental health, we can help to build a more informed, compassionate, and proactive approach to mental wellness. Whether you are a mental health professional, a policymaker, or simply someone who cares about the well-being of yourself and others, there is always more to learn and discover in the pursuit of mental health and resilience.

References

1.   Solomon, A. (2015). The Noonday Demon: An Atlas of Depression. Scribner.
2.   van der Kolk, B. (2015). The Body Keeps the Score: Brain, Mind, and Body in the Healing of Trauma. Penguin Books.
3.   Watters, E. (2010). Crazy Like Us: The Globalization of the American Psyche. Free Press.
4.   Metzl, J. M. (2010). The Protest Psychosis: How Schizophrenia Became a Black Disease. Beacon Press.
5.   Harris, R. (2008). The Happiness Trap: How to Stop Struggling and Start Living. Trumpeter.
6.   National Institute of Mental Health. (2021). Mental Health Information. https://www.nimh.nih.gov/health/topics/index.shtml
7.   Substance Abuse and Mental Health Services Administration. (2021). Publications and Resources. https://www.samhsa.gov/resources
8.   National Alliance on Mental Illness. (2021). Research and Innovation. https://www.nami.org/Learn-More/Research-and-Innovation
9.   World Health Organization. (2021). Mental Health. https://www.who.int/health-topics/mental-health

Glossary of Mental Health Terms

As we have explored throughout this book, the field of mental health is vast and complex, encompassing a wide range of conditions, treatments, and approaches. For those who are new to the world of mental health, or who are seeking to deepen their understanding of key concepts and terminology, it can be helpful to have a glossary of common mental health terms on hand. In this section, we will provide definitions and explanations for some of the most important and frequently used terms in the field of mental health.

One of the most fundamental terms in mental health is "mental illness" or "mental disorder." These terms refer to a wide range of conditions that affect a person's thinking, feeling, mood, and behavior. Mental illnesses can range from mild to severe, and can impact a person's ability to function in daily life. Some common examples of mental illnesses include depression, anxiety disorders, bipolar disorder, and schizophrenia [1].

Another important term in mental health is "diagnosis." A diagnosis is the process of identifying and labeling a specific mental health condition based on a person's symptoms, history, and other factors. Mental health professionals use standardized diagnostic criteria, such as the Diagnostic and Statistical Manual of Mental Disorders (DSM) or the International Classification of Diseases (ICD), to make diagnoses [2]. Receiving a diagnosis can be an important step in accessing appropriate treatment and support.

"Treatment" is another key term in mental health, referring to the various interventions and approaches used to manage and alleviate the symptoms of mental illness. Treatment can take many forms, including medication, psychotherapy, and other evidence-based practices. The goal of treatment is to help individuals with mental health conditions achieve remission, improve their quality of life, and prevent relapse [3].

One common form of treatment in mental health is "psychotherapy," also known as "talk therapy" or "counseling." Psychotherapy involves meeting with a trained mental health professional to discuss one's thoughts, feelings, and behaviors, and to develop coping strategies and solutions to problems. There are many different types of psychotherapy, including cognitive-behavioral therapy (CBT), dialectical behavior therapy (DBT), and psychodynamic therapy, each with its own approach and focus [4].

Another important aspect of mental health is "recovery," which refers to the process of managing and overcoming the challenges associated with mental illness. Recovery is a highly individualized process that involves developing hope, self-determination, and a sense of purpose and meaning in life. Recovery often involves a combination of treatment, support, and personal growth and development [5].

"Stigma" is another key term in mental health, referring to the negative attitudes, beliefs, and discrimination that often surround mental illness. Stigma can take many forms, including labeling, stereotyping, and social exclusion, and can be a significant barrier to seeking help and achieving recovery. Efforts to reduce stigma and promote mental health awareness and acceptance are an important part of the larger mental health movement [6].

"Resilience" is another important concept in mental health, referring to the ability to adapt and bounce back from adversity and stress. Resilience is not a fixed trait, but rather a set of skills and strategies that can be developed and strengthened over time. Building resilience can involve developing a positive outlook, cultivating social connections and support, and engaging in self-care and stress management practices [7].

"Self-care" is another term that is often used in the context of mental health, referring to the various activities and practices that individuals can engage in to promote their own well-being and manage stress. Self-care can take many forms, including exercise, relaxation techniques, healthy eating, and engaging in hobbies and activities that bring joy and fulfillment [8].

"Mindfulness" is another term that has gained increasing attention in the field of mental health in recent years. Mindfulness refers to the practice of paying attention to the present moment with openness, curiosity, and non-judgment. Mindfulness practices, such as meditation and yoga, have been shown to have a range of mental health benefits, including reducing stress and anxiety, improving mood, and enhancing overall well-being [9].

Finally, "mental health parity" is an important term in the world of mental health policy and advocacy. Mental health parity refers to the idea that mental health services should be covered by insurance at the same level as physical health services. Despite progress in recent years, many insurance plans still do not provide adequate coverage for mental health treatment, leading to significant barriers to access and care [10].

These are just a few of the many important terms and concepts in the field of mental health. By developing a shared language and understanding of these key ideas, we can work together to promote greater awareness, acceptance, and support for those affected by mental health conditions. Whether you are a mental health professional, a policymaker, or simply someone who cares about the well-being of yourself and others, familiarity with these terms can be a valuable tool in navigating the complex and ever-evolving landscape of mental health.

References

1. National Alliance on Mental Illness. (2021). Mental Health Conditions. https://www.nami.org/Learn-More/Mental-Health-Conditions

2. American Psychiatric Association. (2013). Diagnostic and Statistical Manual of Mental Disorders (5th ed.). https://doi.org/10.1176/appi.books.9780890425596

3. National Institute of Mental Health. (2021). Mental Health Medications. https://www.nimh.nih.gov/health/topics/mental-health-medications/

4. American Psychological Association. (2021). Different approaches to psychotherapy. https://www.apa.org/topics/psychotherapy/approaches

5. Substance Abuse and Mental Health Services Administration. (2021). Recovery and Recovery Support. https://www.samhsa.gov/find-help/recovery

6. Corrigan, P. W., & Watson, A. C. (2002). Understanding the impact of stigma on people with mental illness. World Psychiatry, 1(1), 16-20. https://www.ncbi.nlm.nih.gov/pmc/articles/PMC1489832/

7. American Psychological Association. (2021). Building your resilience. https://www.apa.org/topics/resilience

8. National Institute of Mental Health. (2021). Caring for Your Mental Health. https://www.nimh.nih.gov/health/topics/caring-for-your-mental-health/

9. Hofmann, S. G., Sawyer, A. T., Witt, A. A., & Oh, D. (2010). The effect of mindfulness-based therapy on anxiety and depression: A meta-analytic review. Journal of Consulting and Clinical Psychology, 78(2), 169-183. https://doi.org/10.1037/a0018555

10. National Alliance on Mental Illness. (2021). What is Mental Health Parity? https://www.nami.org/Your-Journey/Individuals-with-Mental-Illness/Understanding-Health-Insurance/What-is-Mental-Health-Parity